D0178017

NTAE Á

HAPPY FOOD

Niklas Ekstedt
& Henrik Ennart

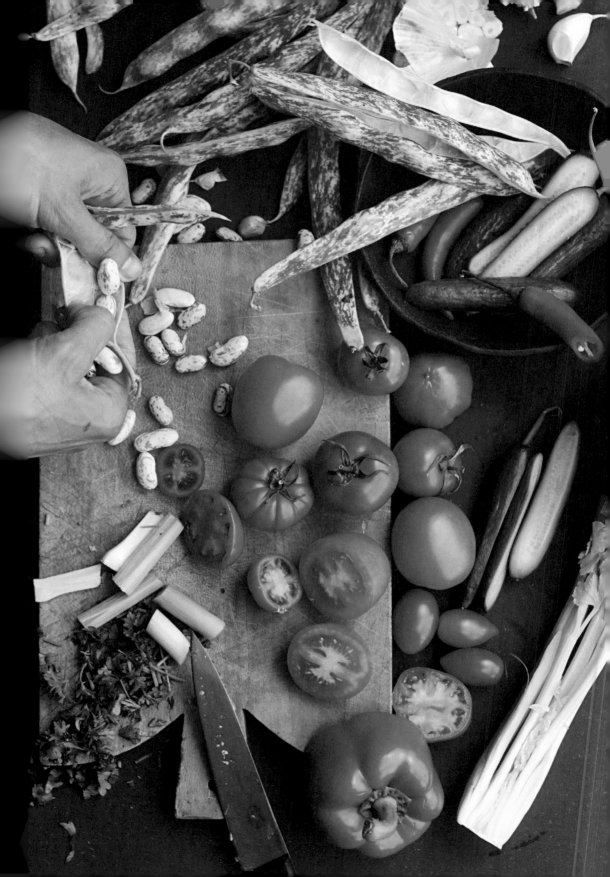

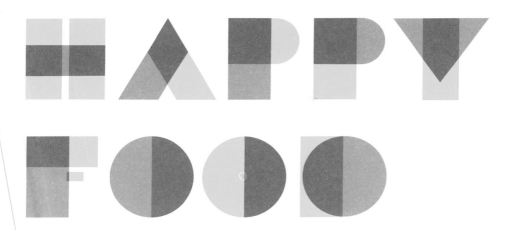

HAPPY FOOD

Niklas Ekstedt
& Henrik Ennart
How eating well can
lift your mood and
bring you joy

Photography: David Loftus

Design and illustration: Katy Kimbell

A.

CONTENTS

PART 1. THE GUT AND THE BRAIN – AND HOW EVERYTHING IS CONNECTED

Part 2. PRESENTING: SUPERFOODS

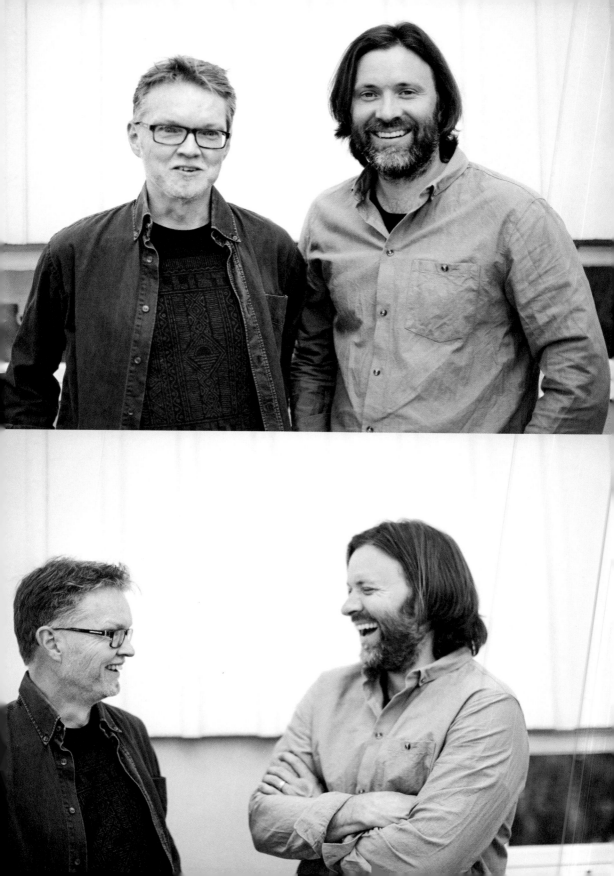

Foreword

This book has changed our lives. It could easily change yours too. Despite the fact that both Niklas and I, Henrik, have devoted the majority of our adult lives to food and how it affects us, working on *Happy Food* has forced us to re-examine everything we thought we knew.

This has been a real game changer.

Even when the food debate has been at its peak, we have long felt that a major, important piece of the puzzle was missing. The bits had never really fitted together properly. Now that missing piece is in place.

Insights into how food affects our gut flora have already cast new light on some of our most common diseases. What we describe in this book is the next revolution.

In early August 2017, I was the only journalist to take part in the first international expert conference entirely devoted to discussing the latest research into how food affects mental health. It was held in the town of Bethesda, near Washington, and brought together leading researchers from universities across the world.

The conclusions reported were clear. According to solid research, the same sugar-rich industrial food that has caused global epidemics of obesity and diabetes, and exponentially increased gluten intolerance, stomach and bowel diseases, is contributing ever more to the current rise of mental illness. At the same time it is becoming ever clearer what kind of food can put everything right.

This is the revolution that we want to describe in *Happy Food*.

FACT: Many people need to be healthier. In 2017 depression was classified by the World Health Organization (WHO) as the second most important global cause of disability. More than 320 million people around the world are affected and the disease is becoming increasingly common. Every fifth person is affected by depression at some point in their lives.

You are what you eat

The food on your plate affects not only your body but also your brain. As well as improving your mood and sharpening your mind, it also works as a treatment for anxiety and severe depression.

Your large intestine, or colon, is like a tank reactor, where the contents ferment and simmer. It produces hormones and signal substances that control your emotions. It's really no coincidence that the gut is sometimes called "the second brain".

New research shows that gut bacteria don't merely affect our body weight, chronic bowel diseases, diabetes, cardiovascular diseases, Parkinson's, Alzheimer's, anxiety, depression and autism. They also affect how we feel and how fresh and alert we are in our everyday lives. They even help shape our personality.

Have you heard of the biological revolution, which is predicted to be bigger than the IT revolution and could be one of the most important issues in this century? The revolution that will consign some of our most feared diseases to the dustbin, and perhaps even help us fight ageing itself?

It's already here!

More than half of all research ever done on gut flora has been published in the last two years. New findings are being published almost every hour. And, if anything, that rate is actually increasing.

We want to guide you through the latest findings and emphasise broad-based research into how the gut can help your brain.

We will introduce you to your own gut bacteria and explain what food is best both for you and your tiny companions, and also how, just like you, the residents in your basement can be affected by stress and are healthier if they get regular rest and exercise.

We look at the similarities between the Mediterranean diet, Scandinavian and Japanese food and explain why barley, beans and Jerusalem artichokes are party food for your gut flora, but also how you need more than this to create a healthy gut.

We explain why colours, scents and tastes aren't merely for your eyes, nose and taste buds and how your gut flora can become your best defence against toxins and fungal attacks.

Food regulates how we feel, and it does so here and now. Within 24 hours, the food you've just eaten will have altered the flora of bacteria that live in your guts in a way that it is now possible to measure. These are changes that we can already begin to link to increased or reduced risk of a range of diseases, including effects on your mental well-being. This new knowledge forces us to reassess a number of old lessons and preconceived ideas.

For the last 15 years, as a science journalist at the *Svenska Dagbladet* newspaper, in books and on TV, I have examined the food industry and covered research into food, health and ageing. Back in the early 2000s I was reporting on gut bacteria, fibre,

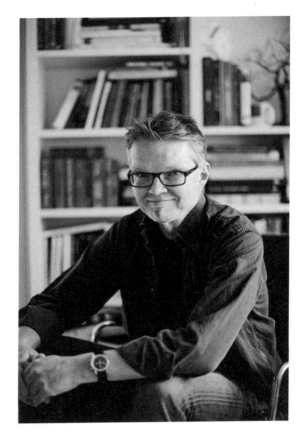

sugar, omega-3 and its connection to hyperactivity and attention deficit disorders. In several series, I have presented the link between chronic inflammation simmering under the surface and mental illness.

Niklas Ekstedt is one of Sweden's leading star chefs. His cutting-edge expertise in cooking and in-depth knowledge of ingredients and traditional culinary skills have made it possible to transform the latest scientific findings into delicious and innovative dishes that everyone can prepare. Niklas is one of the people who introduced Scandinavian food onto the international stage.

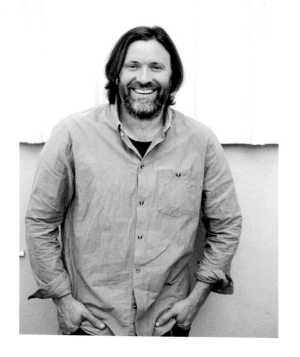

Happy Food contains 38 recipes for food that's both tasty and healing, not merely good for the body but also for the soul.

The book is based on wide-ranging and independent fact collection. We have no patents or research careers to defend, and have therefore been able to interview different experts who aren't always in agreement with each other, in a humble and balanced manner.

But many research results speak for themselves. And if it's possible to serve food that gives us a healthier mind, which makes us more cheerful and can even help counteract mental illnesses, then it's time to abandon any neutrality. Because this is something we must all embrace immediately! Anything else would be irresponsible. Particularly as good food is a cheap alternative to medicine – and lacks any nasty side-effects.

Around 2,500 years ago, the father of medicine, Hippocrates, said, "Let food be thy medicine" – but this doesn't mean that food has to taste like medicine too!

Nor that healthy food has to be blended in a mixer!

The secret is that food which creates a sound, flourishing and multicultural micro-landscape in your gut must be as varied as your gut flora. This type of food can be easy to prepare and tastes really great.

We call it Happy Food!

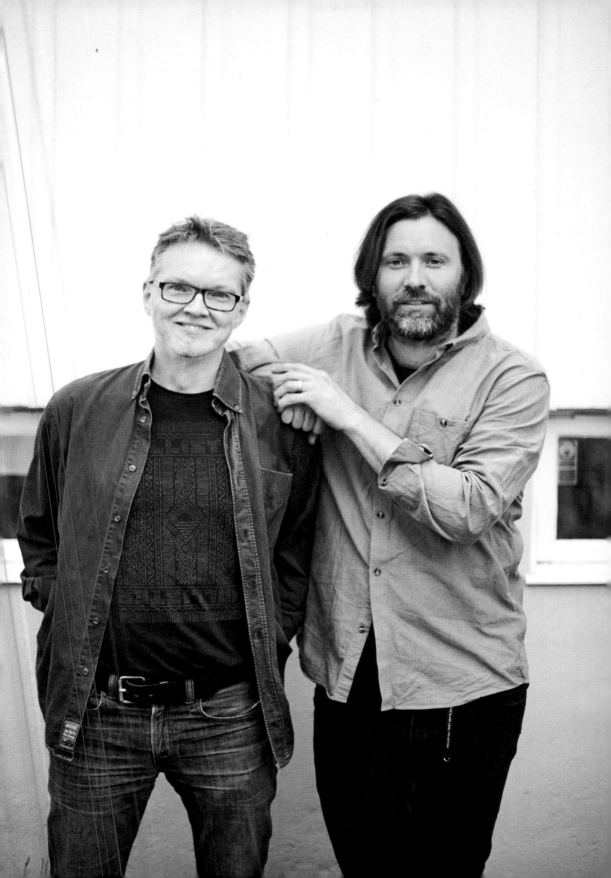

THE GUT AND THE BRAIN

— AND HOW EVERY- THING IS CONNECTED

Part 1.

Everything starts in the gut. A gut feeling is something humans have always believed in. We get butterflies in our stomach when we fall in love, feel sick to our stomach when we're unfairly treated and go on gut feeling when we make instinctive decisions.

In recent years, we have begun to realise that the link between gut and brain is far stronger than we had previously thought.

So let's have a closer look at Gut Feeling 2.0.

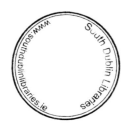

WHY SETTLE FOR POOR HEALTH WHEN YOU DON'T HAVE TO?

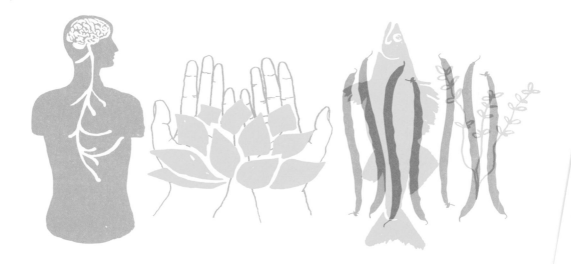

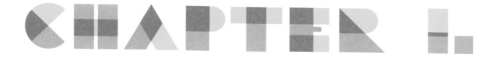

CHAPTER 1.

Your second brain

Your gut bacteria weigh 1.4 kg. About the same as your brain. There's an enormous number of them – around 40 trillion, according to new calculations – and every gram of mucus covering the walls of your colon contains billions of bacteria.

Today, we are starting to understand that, together with the food we eat, these residents of our guts directly affect our mental health. If we treat them well, they won't merely help us to become more stress-resistant, alert, happy and harmonious. A rapidly growing body of research also shows a direct link between the condition of gut flora and depression and other mental illnesses.

Your gut bacteria have more cells and genetic material than the rest of your whole body. It almost doesn't matter what you put in your mouth, there's a type of gut bacteria that specialises in attacking or breaking down that particular item and transforming it into something your body needs and can absorb.

As we'll see in more detail in a later chapter, the gut bacteria are also very closely linked to the central nervous system and a number of other channels in direct contact with your head. The gut bacteria are quite simply an

extension of your brain. Or perhaps it's the other way around. Because they were actually here billions of years before us, and our brains developed in their environment.

You couldn't survive for long without many of the things that your friendly gut bacteria do for you. They cobble together vitamins and hormones that help us to be healthy. They protect us against environmental toxins and yeast invasions. But that's not all. Every signal substance that your brain uses can be manufactured by your gut bacteria in their microscopic workshops.

Your gut flora is an ecosystem that reflects your environment. If the diversity of species in the environment around you is depleted, if the environment is full of toxins and you're inhaling exhaust fumes, if you're constantly stressed and eating a repetitive diet, it will unavoidably affect the life inside you. Any imbalances that occur in your gut flora are propagated throughout your entire body and put a strain on your mental health. Thanks to research into gut flora, we have now finally started to understand how all of this works. And it has suddenly become obvious that we are part of a greater whole. For us to be really happy, the world around us must be healthy and happy too!

How can it be that this is entirely new knowledge that we hadn't suspected until very recently?

In the early 2000s when researchers mapped the human genome, they developed a technique for quickly analysing genes. Less than ten years ago, these new techniques were first used to map the human microbiota.

This is an expression that covers bacteria, viruses, yeasts and what are now known as archaea, but in practice researchers haven't yet been able to investigate more than just the bacteria, which are by far the most populous of these micro-organisms. So we won't have the entire picture before the interplay between all of these microbes has been completely investigated. It's an enormous job.

Researchers were once forced to cultivate bacteria in their laboratories. As well as being time-consuming, it simply wasn't possible for many of the bacteria – which normally live in the oxygen-poor environment of the colon – to be cultivated in this way.

The few exceptions that could be cultivated in the lab included lactic acid bacteria such as lactobacillus casei etc. You no doubt recognise these from live yoghurts.

Lactic acid bacteria undoubtedly have an important role to play, but in terms of research they are a thing of the past. Now, completely different bacteria are being studied, which are both more common and more important in the gut.

The number of different species that live in the gut is one of the very clearest signs of good (or poor) health. The more species, the better. Pretty much every disease, of both body and soul, is associated with a lower number of species in the gut.

One important new insight is that some of our gut bacteria are threatened by extinction.

The same thing applies to normal ageing. We have the fewest species in our gut when we are born, but we are quickly supplied with lactobacillus and bifidobacteria from our mother's breasts, skin and vagina. These bacteria quickly create a pleasant environment for other species to establish themselves.

The number of species present in the gut then increases quickly to reach a peak in the young adult, before gradually reducing throughout the rest of our lives. And as this takes place, many other functions deteriorate, including our immune system and our ability to absorb nutrition from our food.

One conceivable strategy for slowing ageing is therefore to try to prevent the elimination of the gut bacteria.

The warning that our gut bacteria are as threatened by extinction as many vulnerable species of plants and animals came from researchers who had travelled around the world and analysed faeces samples from indigenous populations.

While in the Western world we generally have between 800 and 1,000 different types of bacteria in the gut, people living in a traditional way have a much more varied gut flora, with up to 1,600 species. And these are often different species too. Many of the bacteria found in indigenous populations are completely absent in the Western world.

The quantity of gut bacteria during a lifetime

These findings reflect the fact that many of us in the West now eat a very repetitive diet. If you look around in a supermarket, there are thousands of products – but if you read the labels you realise that many of them are filled with the same few ingredients, such as wheat, sugar and corn. For indigenous populations, it's exactly the opposite. Hardly any products, but lots of different ingredients.

Twelve plant species and five animal species constitute three quarters of all food on the planet.

Most common plants in order:
Sugar cane
Maize
Rice
Wheat
Potatoes
Soya beans
Cassava
Tomatoes
Bananas
Onion
Apples
Grapes

The most common animals (meat):
Pigs
Chickens
Cattle
Sheep
Goats

Out of the roughly 300,000 edible plant species on our planet, we in the Western world use at most 200. According to a major survey carried out in 2016, three quarters of all food consumed on the Earth comes from just twelve plant and five animal species. You can probably think of most of these yourself: wheat, corn, soya, rice, palm oil…

Many bacteria appear to be quite fussy about their food. If they don't get their favourite dish, they quite simply skip their meals. In other words, our original gut flora consisted of many different types of bacteria that liked the ingredients we no longer eat. Certainly, some of our bacteria are extremely patient and can lie idle in the gut for a long time waiting for a feast, but eventually they give up and die off.

And for every extinct bacterium, the imbalance in the gut's ecosystem increases – and your resistance against stress and infections reduces at the same rate. Perhaps you feel as though your head is constantly shrouded in fog.

Because not only have ingredients become fewer, they have also become more processed.

But the wheat eaten around the Mediterranean since Antiquity – as a moderate addition to an extremely varied menu – has very little in common with today's finely ground wheatmeal.

For many people today, 'wheat' is almost a dirty word because of its gluten content and high GI.

When wheat grain is no longer eaten whole or roughly crushed, but transformed into a fine dust in modern mills with steel rollers, almost all of the nutritious vitamins and minerals disappear. All that's left is the energy-rich starch, which is absorbed by the small intestine. For that, we don't need gut bacteria as we can manage with our own enzymes.

In the small intestine, flour contributes to rapid blood sugar fluctuations – and mood swings – and ultimately, to the epidemic of Type 2 diabetes. The coarse grains never reach the colon, where the husk once provided food for hungry gut bacteria. In other words, the problem is primarily related to particle size rather than the grain in itself.

So this is a problem of several stages. First the wheat grain has changed dramatically through cultivation, so that today it contains fewer minerals and vitamins and more protein in the form of gluten. In the next stage, the method of grinding the grain itself has given it an entirely new destructive function in the human body. Finally, our own gut flora is depleted because it doesn't receive any fibre to live on.

In the same way, pretty much everything we eat has been transformed from fibre-rich to easily digested and has been stripped of its minerals, vitamins, flavonoids and other healthy substances. In their place you instead risk ingesting traces of pesticides or mycotoxins that your already embattled gut flora find difficult to resist.

The consequences are catastrophic. Regardless of which illness breaks out, you can be sure that your gut flora will be decimated.

The good news is that you can do something about it. You can build your own happiness!

Like Downton Abbey: "All the action takes place in the basement"

"If you eat a varied diet, you can maintain a varied gut flora and this can really help your digestive health, your brain health and your entire immune system," says world-leading researcher John Cryan, who is Head Investigator for the Microbiome Institute at the University of Cork.

John Cryan's interest in gut flora arose when he was researching stress. One early experiment showed that stressful experiences in young mice had a lifelong impact on the animals' gut flora.

In a series of later experiments, his group has demonstrated how mice with an entirely sterile gut have a stronger stress reaction and impaired anxiety regulation. This meant that they could no longer assess risks and social situations. In other words, they develop typical symptoms of autism.

"We have strong evidence today for saying that the gut flora can be linked to autism. We can even change a mouse's personality and behaviour by transplanting its gut flora. We can transform neurotic mice into relaxed ones and back again. But at the moment we're only at the stage of animal testing. We need more research to show similar links in humans," says John Cryan.

He is convinced that such results are only a question of time and resources.

John Cryan and other researchers have also been able to demonstrate that the gut flora can cause structural changes in the brain. These include effects on the secretion of myelin in the frontal lobe.

Myelin is a substance that forms an insulating layer around the nerve cells in the brain. Myelin shortages are associated with neurological diseases such as MS and even cognitive impairment in older people. In healthy people, myelin contributes to reducing energy leakage and keeping the brain sharp and alert. We have most myelin as young adults, but as is often the case, enough is as good as a feast. Too much myelin is linked to high levels of risk seeking, asocial behaviour and even schizophrenia.

Researchers are now working to stabilise secretion of myelin at an appropriate level by adjusting the gut flora.

Even the substance BDNF (brain derived neurotrophic factor), which contributes to improving memory and learning, increases with a healthy gut flora. This substance is sometimes called "brain fertiliser", because it protects the connections between brain cells and helps to create new ones. BDNF is also stimulated by exercise.

"We're terribly snobbish when it comes to the brain and how complicated it is," says John Cryan with a laugh.

John Cryan sees major similarities between how psychiatry has ignored the body and only worried about the brain, and the popular TV series *Downton Abbey*.

"Two groups live together in the same house, but the inhabitants of the upper floors try to completely ignore the ones downstairs. But it's in the basement that all the important things happen."

Stanford researchers Justin and Erica Sonnenburg are among those who investigated indigenous people in the Amazon and discovered that they have many gut bacteria completely unknown to us.

Back in their own laboratory, they fed mice a normal, fibre-poor Western diet, and the animals' gut flora was dramatically reduced. This was even passed down to their children and grandchildren. For four mouse generations.

The conclusion is that we can restore our gut flora as long as we have some bacteria left, but what we have lost can be lost for good, regardless of how much fibre we eat. It also means that what we do now can have an impact on our own grandchildren's grandchildren's digestive health.

This insight reverses almost everything we have learned about food and health.

We should also question diets based on the complete exclusion of particular ingredients, particularly those rich in fibre that can provide food for our gut bacteria.

These extreme diets, where we completely avoid such fibre, can even reduce the number of species in our own gut, ultimately making us less healthy!

Does this even apply to intermittent fasting or fasting consistently for a week? Probably not, if it's limited to shorter periods and if you generally eat a varied and fibre-rich diet. Fasting also has many other positive effects.

Does this also apply to a gluten-free diet? Yes, more probably, and there are studies that indicate this. For those who can't tolerate gluten and suffer from coeliac disease, of course there's no option but to completely avoid these foods. However, if you suffer from more general symptoms, avoiding fibre and coarse whole grains can instead lead to more depleted gut flora and symptoms that actually deteriorate.

So what was our original gut flora like? The Sonnenburgs describe our Western gut flora as resembling the site of an aeroplane crash where accident investigators are trying to fit the pieces back together. Many pieces are missing and there are lots of gaps.

And this is the catastrophic condition of the gut flora in many otherwise healthy people in the Western world. For those suffering from a chronic bowel disease, but also for those who are stressed or suffering from burnout or many mental illnesses, the gaps are even greater.

Because the Western lifestyle has spread rapidly over the world, it's extremely urgent that researchers seek out and investigate indigenous populations before they too have succeeded in destroying their gut flora with fibre-poor junk food.

It isn't merely the number of different types of gut bacteria that vary. Indigenous populations also have a different balance, dominated by bacteria that are usually associated with good health.

These are the type of gut bacteria that flourish when you eat a lot of wild, fibre-rich plants, fish and game.

The Hazda people, who live in Tanzania near what is generally known as the cradle of humanity in the Great Rift Valley, are one of the groups most likely to provide clues about what our original gut flora was like before agriculture became widespread.

The Hazda eat meat from game, fruit, berries and root vegetables which are so fibre-rich that they have to spit out balls of the toughest fibres. The menu also includes millet seed, the African seed teff, durra, which is a grass seed, together with pulses, herbs and leafy vegetables.

In total, it is estimated that they eat 100–150 grams of fibre a day. That's about ten times as much as we eat in the Western world, and five times as much as nutrition authorities recommend.

The consequence is therefore that our gut flora is reduced.

This is unfortunate, because our gut bacteria are designed for dealing with and breaking down nutrients and protecting us from unwelcome visitors. The reduced defences thus contribute to both food allergies and chronic diseases. Increased gluten intolerance

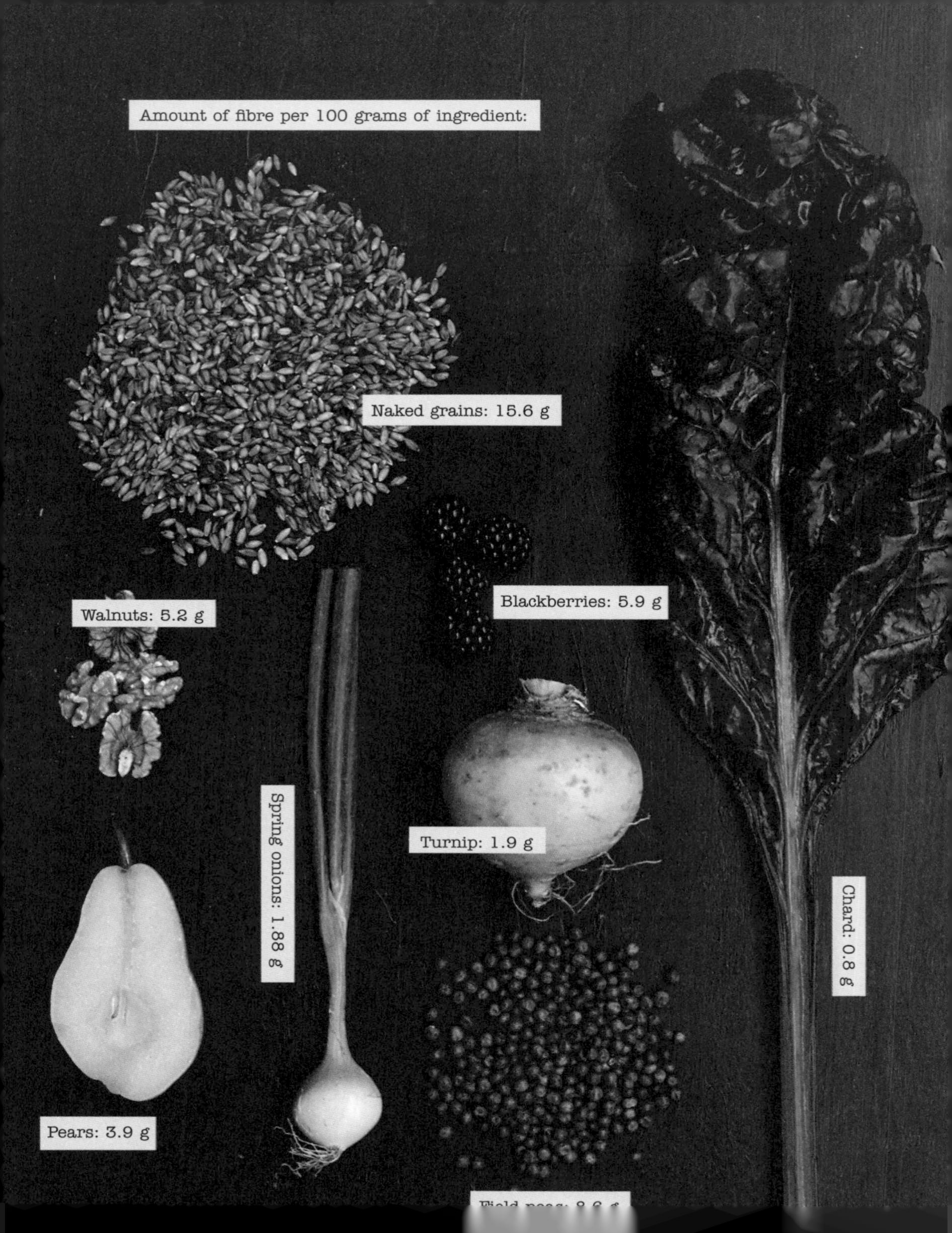

Amount of fibre per 100 grams of ingredient:

Naked grains: 15.6 g

Walnuts: 5.2 g

Blackberries: 5.9 g

Spring onions: 1.88 g

Turnip: 1.9 g

Chard: 0.8 g

Pears: 3.9 g

Field peas: 8.6 g

is also believed to be a consequence. And finally, it also affects our brain and general well-being.

Indigenous peoples have a gut flora that's perfectly adapted to the food eaten locally, which can vary significantly. People are omnivores – experts at subsisting on wildly varying ingredients – and we can thank our gut bacteria for this.

Such a local adaptation of gut flora also applies to the Inuit in Greenland, who only eat plant fibre for short periods of the year. Instead they developed a gut flora adapted to fermented food and animal fibre, including from the animal's skin, which formed part of the diet. A favourite dish is shark or seal, which is buried in a gravel pit in the sterile landscape and then left to ferment for three months. The key seems to be perfect adaptation to local conditions.

Just like in all ecosystems, sensitivity increases when the number of species falls. In the natural environment, birds and other animals have more difficulty finding food when insects and plants disappear around large fields of single crops. Many species are specialised and dependent on each other, but more species increase the chances that another will fill the void. With few species, the imbalances increase, which ultimately leads to a sudden and complete collapse.

But you can create a peaceful, multicultural society in your own digestive system.

It's when differences are encouraged, increased variation is recognised and none of our more than 1,000 different species of bacteria is permitted to dominate and take over, that our internal ecosystem has a chance to achieve equilibrium. This is how we maximise the possibility of keeping ourselves healthy and feeling good.

The researchers we have spoken to agree that food is the most important factor in affecting our gut bacteria, but of course there are other aspects of our lifestyle that have great impact.

These include smoking (of course, as always), exercise, sleep and eating at fixed times, but also Caesarean sections, breastfeeding and courses of antibiotics. There is also reason to raise a warning finger regarding our fetish for cleanliness and excessive use of antibacterial products.

The gut-brain axis — how bacteria control our emotions

Regardless of how imbalances occur in the digestive system, they can have repercussions on both the human body and brain. Researchers have been amazed at the strength of the link between the gut and the brain. To understand how food can be so important in making us feel good, we need to look in more detail at how the two collaborate.

We often justify fast and impulsive decisions by blaming them on gut feeling. But these aren't actually unfounded decisions. "Gut feeling" is the result of a swarm of signals sent from the gut to the brain. The digestive tract even has its own nervous system, which is why it's sometimes called "the second brain".

The brain in the gut is an independent part of our autonomous nervous system, which regulates many processes in the body without us having to think about it. So the gut doesn't have an intelligent brain that can think outside the box. Only the brain in our head can do this.

The nervous system that surrounds the gut contains more than 500 million nerve cells. That's as many as in the entire spinal column. In recent years, researchers have worked intensively to understand why we need so many and what all of these nerve cells actually do.

This burgeoning area of research is called the gut-brain axis. And one thing is clear: gut bacteria play an extremely important role!

The nerve cells around the gut are there simply to capture what all of our trillions of gut bacteria are doing. They report how many calories, minerals and vitamins have arrived in the gut, so that the brain knows when it will need topping up.

Everything is registered and carefully noted by the nerve cells around the gut, which then report the information to the brain. This takes place via a number of parallel paths:

The vagus nerve: There is hardly anything that takes place in the gut, or elsewhere in the body, that the vagus nerve is not aware of. It's one of the body's largest nerves, and represents a kind of directly connected high-speed link between the gut and the brain. Constant two-way communication takes place via this nerve, but nine-tenths of this communication is sent up to the brain from the gut cells. The brain then sends out instructions based on the data collected by its bacterial spies in the gut.

The immune defence system: The importance of the gut bacteria in our immune systems cannot be underestimated. They actually form a key part of our immune system. Our resident bacteria can themselves attack and throw out unwelcome guests such as yeasts, toxic substances and gastroenteritis bacteria. They can alert our immune system and even act as

supervisors to ensure it works correctly. But if imbalances occur, the gut bacteria can also react incorrectly, sending out the wrong orders and actually causing chronic inflammation.

The hormone system: Up to 95% of the hormones that control processes in our bodies are manufactured by or in collaboration with the gut bacteria. For example, this includes the hormones that regulate happiness, stress, hunger and satiety. Their signals to the brain are among those transported by the vagus nerve.

Antioxidants: Several of the substances created in the gut have antioxidant effects and protect the body's cells from being attacked and broken down by oxygen free radicals. This process is called oxidative stress, but this is only a more elegant way of explaining that the fat in the cells starts to go rancid, just like butter does if left out on the kitchen counter. You can also compare it to when a car rusts. The antioxidants are the rustproofing agent.

Lymph: One explanation why psychiatry treats the brain as separate from the rest of the body is what's known as the blood-brain barrier, which prevents unwanted guests from entering the brain. Even though many signal substances are manufactured in the gut, it was not previously understood how they could get from there into the brain. Today we know that such contacts can take place by various means, including an entirely unknown system that allows lymph to pass into and out of the central nervous system.

Now that researchers have lifted the lid on our gut flora, it's obvious that almost everything we learned previously about food and health must be seen in a new light. In some cases, this will lead to a radical reassessment of previously accepted truths. In other areas, it may turn out that the gut bacteria should be seen as just one more piece of information. Important overall, but not crucial viewed in isolation. Regardless of the conclusion, the world will never be the same again.

Our gut flora has been an extremely hot topic in recent years among researchers, and a constantly recurring theme in top scientific journals such as *Nature, Cell and Science*.

But in parallel with this, the same journals have drawn attention to another major breakthrough made by another category of researchers, namely those interested in the connection between food and mental health.

A great deal has happened in recent decades. The knowledge that food and lifestyle could contribute to brain diseases is only 50 years old. The insight that the greatest danger is sugar and trans fats rather than butter and the like has only emerged in the last ten years.

Only five years ago, it was controversial to assert that dementia disorders could be related to Western junk food. And even today, many people would probably be shocked at the statement that a large number of mental illnesses are largely diet-related.

Research unites the two revolutions: the gut flora revolution and that illuminating how food and various nutrients affect the brain and our mental well-being.

Despite the fact that the researchers are coming from two different directions, they have come to the same conclusion, and are now working together.

To better understand their thought patterns, we spoke to one of them: Australian professor Felice Jacka, who is founder and president of the International Society for Nutritional Psychiatry Research.

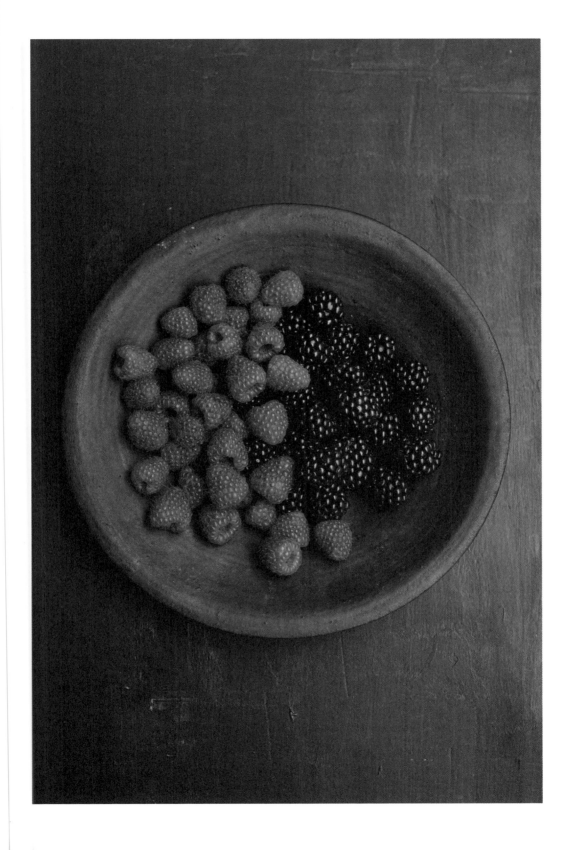

Top researcher: now is the time!

Felice Jacka is the director of the Food and Mood Centre at Deakin University in Melbourne and a world-leading expert in how food affects both our everyday mood swings and severe mental illnesses. In the earthquake of new research that has shaken traditional psychiatry in the last five or six years, Felice Jacka and her colleagues represent a major epicentre, with many results published in respected scientific journals.

Felice:

We know today that there's a link between the food we eat and the epidemic of mental illness. We don't need any more observation studies. There are lots of results like this, and from laboratory testing, and all of them point in the same direction: that food with more vegetables reduces the risk of depression and anxiety and that processed food with a lot of sugar increases the risk. Now it's time to move on and develop and refine diagnosis and treatment methods.

Henrik:

What is it that makes you so convinced?

Felice:

In January 2017, we received the results from the first study ever designed purely to find out whether it was possible to treat severe depression with good food. Among the patients who were given dietary advice there were both those who also received medicine and those who took no medication. It turned out that the effects of dietary advice were much better than treatment with only medication and conversational therapy.

Henrik:
Did it help everyone?

Felice:
No, out of the 56 patients who took part, around one third experienced major improvements. That's a level we've also seen in earlier, simpler studies of anxiety and depression. And it's about the same proportion as feel better when they take medication. There are also indications that the impact of food is even greater on less severe symptoms.

Henrik:
And what did the patients eat?

Felice:
Over a 12-week period, they ate a variant of the Mediterranean diet, with less meat than normal and more vegetables: lots of leafy green vegetables, beans, whole grains, fruit and olive oil. We saw a clear connection between how well they succeeded in changing their eating habits and how much they recovered. It was absolutely fantastic to see.

Henrik:
And what conclusions do you draw from that?

Felice:
That it's high time to start to look at diet as an independent treatment method for depression and anxiety. For me, that's just obvious. We have

a worldwide epidemic of mental illness that's causing enormous suffering and which is costing society a great deal of money. Globally, mental health is the second largest cause of a reduced ability to work. At the same time, we're lacking effective treatment methods. The medications used can lead to severe side-effects, but still only help some people.

In this position, we see from a large number of studies of different types that really fresh food can reduce symptoms dramatically, and if not for all of those affected, at least for a large proportion. Good food is also cheaper than medicine and has no side-effects. Of course we need more and larger studies to confirm our results, but my feeling is that there's no reason at all to delay.

Henrik:
Do you mean that mental illness can be a result of eating poor food?

Felice:
Yes, without any doubt. Of course there are other causes which may be inherited or perceived, but the epidemic of increased mental illness follows in the wake of a Western lifestyle with junk food, stress and too little physical activity. We already know that this is the single most important reason for illness and premature death, even in developing countries. Now we're at the point where we all need to appreciate that the brain isn't separate

from the rest of your body. The increase in mental illness is an expression of exactly the same problems as the epidemics of obesity, diabetes, high blood pressure and high blood fats, but also of digestive problems such as IBS (irritable bowel syndrome) and IBD (inflammatory bowel disease).

Henrik:
What's most important, avoiding junk food or eating healthily?

Felice:
You might think that they're two sides of the same coin, but interestingly we see that these are two different things that complement each other. Junk food with lots of sugar, white flour and bad fats makes us sick. Good food, with lots of fibrous vegetables and antioxidants, makes us healthy.

Henrik:
In one study you've even shown that the brain shrinks from eating junk food.

Felice:
For several years, we've been aware from animal testing that the size of the hippocampus – that's the part of the brain which is associated with learning and memory – can be affected by food in both a positive and negative direction. We were recently able to demonstrate for the first time that this also applies to humans. These findings have since been confirmed by another research group.

In people who had consumed a lot of junk food, such as soft drinks, salty snacks and processed meat, the left hippocampus had a smaller volume, while in those who had eaten lots of vegetables, fruit and fish it was larger in volume.

Henrik:
So if I want to feel better in my soul, it's in the gut that I can find the answer?

Felice:
Yes, many connections that we have seen previously but not understood seem to be explained when we learn more about our gut bacteria. Everything in the human body hangs together. We see that mental illness is linked to what's called metabolic syndrome – in other words, obesity, high blood pressure, high blood fats and diabetes. These conditions often occur in groups and cross-fertilise each other. Often they are driven by chronic inflammation and oxidative stress, and affected by our gut bacteria.

Henrik:
How do these mechanisms work?

Felice:
More than 99% of all of our genes are contained in our bacteria, so to that extent we're more bacteria than human. We used to think that our genes were

crucial. Today we know that we can switch the genes on and off, which is called epigenetics, and that our gut bacteria play a very central role in this. The bacteria have many tasks. Obviously they contribute to breaking down the food we eat, but they're also essential to our immune system, in determining our bodyweight, they manufacture important fatty acids that counteract inflammation, and they also manufacture a large proportion of the hormones and signal substances used by the brain. Every week, new research is published about how this communication works. We don't yet understand it all, but a lot seems to take place via the large vagus nerve that links the gut and the brain.

Henrik:
And is what takes place in the gut just a contributory factor or the primary cause?

Felice:
The food needn't be just something that contributes, it can also be the main cause. At the same time, we see that things like post-traumatic stress, which arises for other reasons, can cause inflammation and imbalances in the gut. People with mental problems, autism and other neuropsychiatric and neurological diseases almost always have problems with their digestive systems. It's a two-way thing and feedback is involved, but the vast

majority of signals go from the gut to the brain. And we can more easily affect the gut flora with the food we eat.

Henrik:
How is the gut flora affected by our lifestyle?

Felice:
For thousands of years, our bodies have developed in symbiosis with our gut flora to function optimally with the food we have eaten. And that food has primarily consisted of plant products combined with fish and wild game. But in very recent years, we've seen an enormous change in what we eat. Above all, we eat far fewer vegetables and much more sugar. And this is completely different from what we ate only a generation ago. This change is creating imbalances in the gut flora. And this has effects that we're now trying to understand better.

Henrik:
How long will it be before we see treatment with food in normal mental healthcare?

Felice:
It should already be taking place, even if there's still a lot more to understand. Yet psychologist training doesn't include a single lesson on nutrition, and there's barely any mention of food during medical training either. There's also some reluctance to apply

31

alternative solutions. We've known for decades that physical activity is effective against depression, but it still hasn't made a breakthrough in normal healthcare except in the odd case.

Henrik:
What can we do?

Felice:
I don't think we can re-train all of our doctors and psychologists, but we can change the recommendations so that a dietician is routinely involved.

Henrik:
So what should we eat to feel good?

Felice:
The strongest scientific evidence is available for the traditional Mediterranean diet, the Japanese diet and a Norwegian/Scandinavian diet that includes a lot of fish.

The common factor is that this is traditional food based on a range of locally produced fresh ingredients.

There's a great deal of evidence that us and our gut bacteria are adapted to the food that our own forefathers ate locally. For example, the Japanese have gut bacteria that break down algae, while people in the rest of the world are lacking these and so it's more difficult for them to break down algae. In other words, we're moving towards a more individual diet, which is adapted to us and our specific conditions.

Henrik:
Is there any space in this diet for eating meat?

Felice:
The crucial thing seems to be to consume lots of fibre of different types.

I thought that red meat would be evil, but our results instead indicate a bell-shaped connection, where small amounts of red meat from grass-fed animals – but not processed meat – are better than none at all. That's in terms of health effects. The fat in grass-fed animals is completely different from the fat in industrially raised animals. Then there are other reasons to avoid eating meat, which I completely understand. But there's always a danger in demonising individual foods. You have to take an overall view.

Through her studies, Australian Felice Jacka came into contact with Norwegian researchers. The collaboration resulted in the fact that some of the world's most important studies of food and mental health are based on data from Norway and the Nordic countries.
Which we think is very lucky!

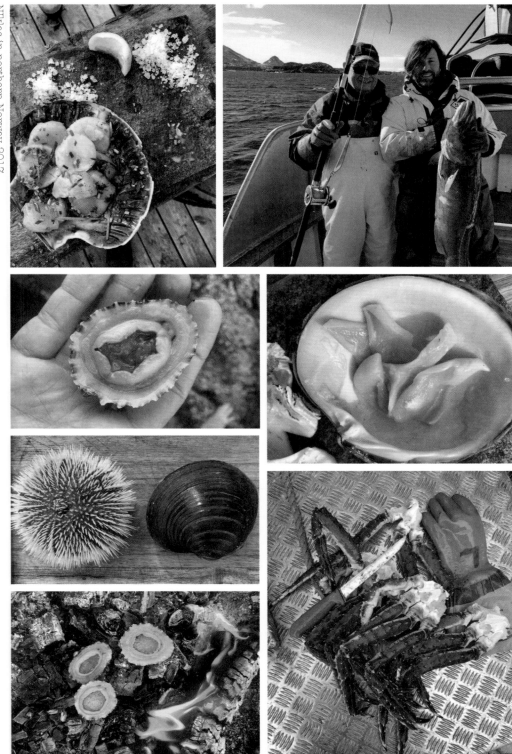

The researchers' route to happy food – year by year

Knowledge about how food affects our mental well-being is ancient, but in recent decades, researchers have used modern scientific methods to take it further, step-by-step.

Here's a very quick overview.

1970

Danish researchers Jørn Dyerberg and Hans Olav Bang travelled to Greenland, where they discovered that the omega-3 fat in the fish-based diet of the indigenous people explained the low mortality from cardiovascular diseases.

1998

In the late 1990s, American researcher Joseph Hibbeln realised that this healthy fish fat also affected the brain and can relieve mental illness and hyperactivity.

2000

Around the turn of the millennium, the vitamin D debate was launched in earnest, and it soon became clear that the sunshine vitamin doesn't merely give stronger bones but can also have an inhibitory effect on depression and other mental illness. What we didn't then know was that, by means of its anti-inflammatory effect, vitamin D contributes to a richer and more well-balanced gut flora.

Reports stated that folate, or vitamin B9, might also have an inhibiting effect on depression. Similar results had been reported in 1991, but had not been made public. Folate is found above all in liver, which we eat less of now than previously – as with all offal – but also in beans and leafy green vegetables.

But attempts to improve mental health by means of individual vitamins and supplements came to a dead end. There seemed to be no connection. A capsule containing omega-3 fats cannot compensate for the damage caused by a generally poor diet with lots of sugar, refined wheat flour, additives and highly processed, hydrogenated oils.

The focus was instead aimed at the effects of complete diets. Now the breakthrough wasn't far off. In 2009 and 2010 three articles were published in prestigious journals that in different ways demonstrated the connection between food and mental health, and how the gut bacteria play a central role.

In the first study, researchers who examined 3,486 Londoners reported that the risk of being affected by depression within five years was significantly increased for those eating sugary, greasy and fried junk food. Conversely, the middle-aged Londoners who instead ate a lot of vegetables were protected against depression.

A new major study soon emerged from Navarra in Spain which showed that the Mediterranean diet seemed to be able to provide protection against depression. A couple of years earlier, researchers had seen that same diet could provide protection against Alzheimer's and Parkinson's diseases.

Now came the study that provided the breakthrough for the Australian research group led by Felice Jacka. It was based on sound Norwegian data from diet surveys and interviews and demonstrated once again that a Western diet with a lot of junk food increases the risk of depression. On the other hand, a Scandinavian, less processed diet with meat, fish, vegetables and whole grains reduces the risk of both depression and anxiety.

In the following years many similar observation studies were published, and finally researchers could carry out what are known as meta-studies, in which the data from a number of sources is brought together and examined. Here too, a strong connection was detected between food and a number of different mental disorders.

The results from the PREDIMED trial were published. This was one of the world's most ambitious dietary studies thus far, and was aimed at investigating the effects of a Mediterranean diet.

Spanish researchers reported that a Mediterranean diet with olive oil and reinforced with nuts provides strong protection against depression for Type 2 diabetics.

Of course many people wondered "why just Type 2 diabetics?" Soon the jigsaw pieces fell into place. Because it has turned out that good eating habits above all help the large group of patients – approximately one third – who, in parallel with mental disorders, suffer from chronic inflammation. Something that affects many Type 2 diabetics.

When researchers around the world then went back and looked at old data with new eyes, they took into account whether or not the patients suffered from chronic inflammation and saw that food had a much clearer effect than had previously been thought.

The first experimental studies that fulfil what researchers normally call *a gold standard* started to deliver results. This is a type of large-scale experiment that can also clear up ambiguities regarding cause and effect. Previously, the majority of results have been based on observational studies, in which researchers retrospectively try to understand what has happened.

In January, an Australian group published the results of the first experimental study designed solely to study the effect of food on severe depression. The question the researchers asked was: what happens if we give dietary advice to patients suffering from the disease?

The result: after 12 weeks, one third of participants had recovered so much that they no longer fulfilled the criteria for the diagnosis.

This is a result comparable to that from many medications, but this time completely without side-effects.

Add to this all the less serious symptoms such as irritation, tiredness and lack of initiative, and it's clear that we should be listening to our gut if we want to be really healthy.

The Australian study, named SMILES, wasn't particularly large and needed to be followed by others. But a further, slightly smaller, experimental study called Helfimed has also come up with almost exactly the same results. In Europe, the much larger MooDFOOD study, sponsored by the European Commission, is expected to start delivering results in 2018. A pilot study presented in summer 2017 gave a clue as to the results: food and the risk of depression go together!

But before we get to grips with all of the uplifting things that we can easily achieve at home in the kitchen, we should get out the magnifying glass and take a closer look at our gut flora, where there has also been enormous progress in the research field. Come along for the ride if you dare!

CRASH COURSE IN
GUT BACTERIA

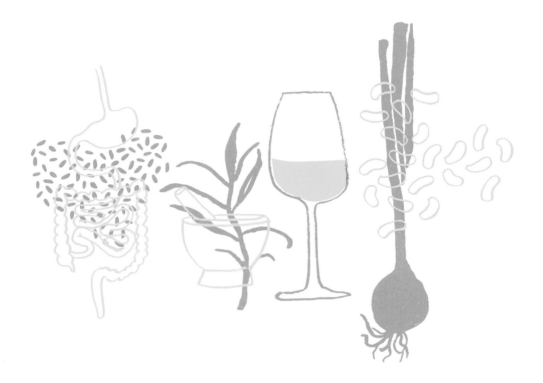

CHAPTER 2.

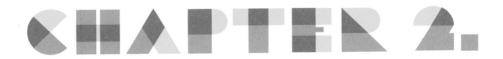

39 What type of gut flora are you? **43** A few key players in the gut flora team – and what they do. **46** Bubbling under.

What type of gut flora are you?

You're either a **Prevotella** or a **Bacteroides**. Probably the latter.

Researchers are working hard to identify the gut flora, and as we've seen, that's a huge job. But the effort will be worthwhile.

The vision is to treat diseases by taking samples and prescribing the bacteria that you are lacking. In the future, this will probably be able to replace many of today's medications.

It's rare for one bacterium to be decisive. Instead, what's involved is a whole ecosystem with hundreds of actors, each of whom must play their part in the cast assembled in your gut.

A bacterium that works well in one context can be transformed into a kind of terrorist in a different environment.

Here are a few things that we know:

Two of the most common types of gut bacteria are called Prevotella and Bacteroides. They don't get on well together at all. When there are many of one, there are few of the other, and vice versa. One of these two usually dominates in the gut, and they then surround themselves with subjects to build entire realms, but most of us can quickly and unsentimentally change side if necessary.

One of these two main types usually represents 10 to 40% of a person's entire gut flora.

Prevotella is common in people who eat a lot of vegetables and fibre. This bacterium usually dominates in those who grew up in the countryside, in areas with a lot of agriculture and in indigenous peoples. Regardless of whether researchers take samples in the countryside in Burkina Faso, South Africa, Malawi, Venezuela or on the Russian steppes, Prevotella is most common.

Prevotella is associated with good health but, just like almost all bacteria, can become aggressive in a damaged and decimated gut flora. Prevotella often works together with the group of useful but sulphurous bacteria that can be recognised by their acrid smell. This is generally a sign of good health.

If you live in Europe or the USA, other industrial countries or in a city, your gut is often ruled by Bacteroides. Bacteroides rapidly gobbles up all available refined carbohydrates, but isn't scared of a quick snack of meat and saturated fat.

This ruler takes power when we stuff ourselves with junk food, and also gains most energy from what we eat so that we become extra fat and round.

It's no wonder that Bacteroides is common in the gut of people who suffer from obesity and a range of chronic and inflammatory diseases.

Once upon a time, Bacteroides was undoubtedly a useful group of reserve bacteria to have on hand in tough times, because they mean that you can eat almost anything and still survive. They are masters at sucking out the last bit of energy from many different sorts of food which would otherwise pass through you and disappear. But when they're allowed to dominate, trouble is on the way.

However, as we've already mentioned, it's more a question of the overall situation than the individual players. Even in the subgroup of Bacteroides, there are more than 50 members and these can also have a positive effect. As just one example, a shortage of one of these bacteria – Bacteroides fragilis – has been shown to be common in cases of autism.

Good teams can be formed in many different ways, so stability and how they find a balance between them is almost as important as the players in themselves.

If the team is unbalanced, individual bacteria take over. This type of imbalance is often seen in cases of disease, both of the body and soul.

Is it possible to measure the specific bacteria in my gut?

Yes, but the research is still in its infancy. And it's very expensive. And it can take a long time. And you need help from world-leading researchers to interpret the results because there are so many members in each bacterial family. And it's actually difficult for the researchers too. So our top tip is to keep a cool head.

Cheaper tests will undoubtedly be available soon, and we already know that the main aim would be to take many samples over a short period, or to follow how your own gut flora changes in real time.

Another future method is bacterial transplantation. A pioneering discovery was made several years ago by a doctor in China. When he investigated one of the country's fattest men, he discovered that this man had almost exclusively only bacteria of Enterobacter type in his gut. These are known for secreting a toxin – endotoxins – which cause inflammation and a lot of other unpleasant things too. No diet had been effective for the fat man, but when the doctor introduced a more well-balanced flora (via the rectum), his weight plummeted.

When the same sorts of Enterobacter that dominated the man's gut flora were introduced into mice, they also became fat. In other words, it was possible to export the fat Chinese man's obesity simply by using a little of his poo!

In a series of much-publicised trials, researchers have investigated how different types of gut flora characterise mice. In one such experiment, faeces from extroverted,

risk-prone mice was transplanted into other rodents who were more introverted and anxious.

The result: the mice changed personality with each other!

Thus far the method has to a large extent been used only on patients who have had their gut flora completely eliminated, roughly like you might format a hard drive and then load new software. But in the future, transplanted faeces is likely to become a treatment method for people to relieve mental problems, but also the treating obesity and all kinds of diseases. It may become as natural to leave a faeces sample with the doctor as to measure your blood pressure.

The idea of faecal transplants is not a new one. In traditional Chinese medicine, something called The Golden Juice was used as early as 300 AD. This was faeces from healthy individuals which was mixed with clay and healing herbs and then buried in an urn for 20 years before being unearthed and served as a tea to patients with diarrhoeal diseases.

Another not very distant future scenario is the possibility of making deposits in a faeces bank before undergoing treatment with antibiotics or radiation. This is already applied in some hospitals in Canada. The idea is to quickly restore your gut flora if it is damaged during treatment.

And imagine if we could make a deposit in a poo bank when we were young and then make withdrawals later in life to replace bacteria that we had lost. Perhaps this would slow down the development of chronic diseases and help us to live longer. Poo may turn out to be the ultimate rejuvenation treatment!

As we mentioned earlier, reduced variety and species diversity in the gut is part of our ageing process. This contributes to imbalances that weaken the immune system. This is known as "inflamm-ageing".

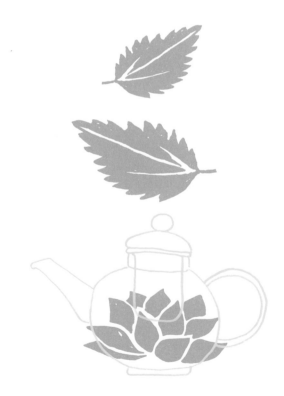

A few key players in the gut flora team – and what they do

While our gut flora varies significantly, there is a core of bacteria that almost everyone carries around within them. At the time of writing, these are completely unknown to most of us. But soon many of them will be on every front page, and in every social media flow about food and health – just like vitamins are today.

If you want to wait until then, you can skip a couple of pages. But if you'd like to get a glimpse into the future, read on!

We used to believe that the majority of gut bacteria were neutral and not really of interest. But as our knowledge has increased, it has become obvious that the importance of the gut flora has been significantly underestimated and that, on the contrary, in many cases it plays a very important role in our health.

While your genes and mine overlap each other to 99.9%, on average only about one sixth of our gut bacteria's genes overlap each other. This not only explains why we react differently to the same food but also why medicines have such an individual effect, and why we don't all have the same resistance to environmental toxins.

So let's get to know the team most often present in your gut.

In the Western world, we usually carry between 800 and 1,000 different types of bacteria in our gut, but around 30 to 40 of these species represent 99% of the total number of bacteria. The most common can be divided into four overall families:

Firmicutes: most common and often represents more than 50%.

Bacteroidetes: up to 40%.

Actinobacteria: up to 20%.

Proteobacteria: up to just over 10%.

In a healthy, stable gut flora, Firmicutes and Bacteroidetes seem to balance each other out. Both families contain friendly and less friendly bacteria.

One clear example of this is the individual bacteria groups Prevotella and Bacteroides, which we mentioned earlier, and which are thought to reflect our eating habits. Prevotella increases if you eat a lot of vegetables, and Bacteroides is associated with Western food. But both of these form part of the parent family of Bacteroidetes.

An increased proportion of Firmicutes is associated with obesity and a Western lifestyle. The total number of Bacteroidetes then usually increases if you lose weight and eat healthily with a lot of vegetables.

It's worth repeating this. We're talking about large families that contain both well-behaved and badly behaved members.

Actinobacteria are very common in soil and contribute to plant decay. In the gut, actinobacteria create stability and are a sign of good health.

In people who suffer from a range of bowel diseases, proteobacteria are often more dominant. As you can imagine from the name, they mostly live on protein.

A compilation was recently carried out of the human microbial core – in other words the gut bacteria that most people have. This doesn't mean that they are greatest in volume, but that they are most common, which means that they are particularly important:

Faecalibacterium prausnitzii (*Firmicutes*): Found in 100% of us. Manufacture butyric acid and other important substances. Anti-inflammatory. Reduced occurrence in the bowel disease IBD, obesity, Crohn's disease and rectal cancer. Reduced quantity linked to both the occurrence and degree of bipolar disorder. Reduces significantly in response to a low fibre diet.

Bifidobacterium (*Actinobacteria*): Found in 99.5% of us. Breaks down carbohydrates. Creates an environment where other friendly bacteria flourish. Common in live yoghurts. Reduces significantly in response to a low fibre diet. Good for short-chain fatty acids, the intestinal mucosa and leaky gut. Reduced occurrence in cases of obesity.

Akkermansia (*Verrucomicrobia*): Found in 96% of all people. Contributes to a healthy gut. Used as a marker for a healthy metabolism. Anti-inflammatory. Reduced occurrence linked to the bowel disease IBD and obesity.

Prevotella melaninogenica (*Bacteroidetes*): Found in 89% of us. Manufactures short-chain fatty acids such as butyric acid. Common in indigenous populations and in response to a diet containing lots of vegetables.

Ruminococcus bromii (*Firmicutes*): Found in 88% of us. An important cornerstone in a healthy gut flora which contributes positive health effects during the breakdown of resistant starch. Reduces in response to a low fibre, low carbohydrate diet.

Bacteroides fragilis (*Bacteroidetes*): Found in 86% of the population. Has an anti-inflammatory effect but can be pathogenic in the case of imbalance. Shortage common in cases of autism.

Roseburia (*Firmicutes*): A group that is often lacking in cases of the bowel disease IBD, ulcerative colitis and IBS. Produces butyric acid. Increased amounts are linked to weight loss and better insulin sensitivity. Reduces in response to a low fibre diet.

Lactobacillus (*Firmicutes*): Common in live yoghurts. Reduces in response to a low fibre diet. Creates a favourable environment in the gut, anti-inflammatory. Reduced occurrence in the case of the bowel disease IBD.

Eubacterium (*Firmicutes*): Key player in the production of short-chain fatty acids. Reduced occurrence in the case of the bowel disease IBD.

Bubbling under

Here are two bacteria that are bubbling under in the gut – in other words two hot names of the future.

Akkermansia muciniphila – the fat eating bacterium

Akkermansia muciniphila affects the metabolism, and the hope is that it will be possible to use the bacterium as a slimming product.

If the gut flora was a football team, this bacterium would be a defensive midfielder, as it gives power and energy to lots of other bacteria in the colon. *Akkermansia muciniphila* also produces a toxin that destroys unwelcome gastroenteritis bacteria.

Studies show that intake of pomegranates, grape pips and cranberries, but also of beans, fish oil and the fibre arabinoxylan that can be found in cereal grains, can be connected to a particularly large increase in the bacterium.

Low incidences associated with a variety of ailments, from the bowel disease IBD to obesity and Type 2 diabetes.

The bacteria eat the intestinal mucus that comes from above and brings with it fibre, and is therefore indirectly positively affected by many different types of fibre.

Faecalibacterium prausnitzii – the super bacterium that loves red wine

Faecalibacterium prausnitzii is the only bacterium that seems to be present in everyone's gut flora. It is also the gut bacterium that has the most genes, which leads to exuberant activity in many different areas. For example, it produces butyric acid and counteracts inflammation. Low levels can be seen in the bowel diseases IBS, IBD, Crohn's disease, coeliac disease and constipation. In a study carried out in the summer of 2017, a shortage of the bacteria was also linked to bipolar disorders – the lower the level, the worse the symptoms of the disease.

News on this bacterium keeps pouring in. Most recently it was reported that it seems to counteract fatty liver disease, hinder the spread of cancer and increase cancer patients' ability to withstand tough treatments.

In one trial where sick patients were placed on a Mediterranean diet and became significantly less ill, higher levels of *Faecalibacterium prausnitzii* were one of the biggest changes in the gut.

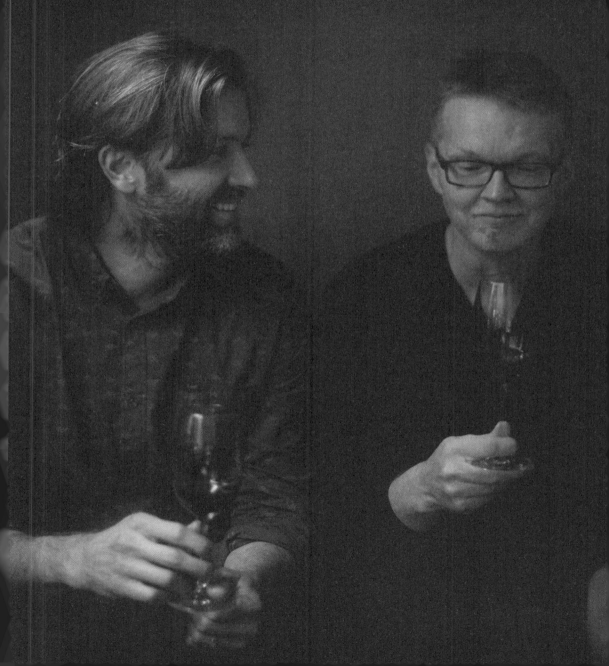

Faecalibacterium prausnitzii enjoys chickpeas and other beans, as well as Jerusalem artichokes and alliums, but also appreciates the phenols in red wine. This may actually be a link that at least partially explains red wine's positive effect on body and soul.

BLOOD SUGAR BLUES FEAT. THE LEAKY GUTS

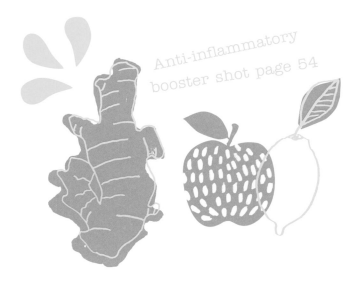

Anti-inflammatory booster shot page 54

CHAPTER B.

Inflammation – a smouldering fire inside you

If you hear the word inflammation, your first thought is probably not about how you feel but instead of a strained, tender and swollen shoulder. Inflammation usually subsides quite quickly.

But sometimes it continues for weeks, months or years and can severely impair your health. It was American heart doctor Paul Ridker who found the first clues to this discovery in the 1990s. He was trying to understand why more than half of his heart patients did not suffer from high cholesterol, as at that time it was the dominant explanation for cardiac diseases.

It turned out that chronic inflammation contributes to atherosclerosis, vascular rigidity, high blood pressure and cardiac and vascular diseases including stroke. In the time since, such chronic inflammation has also proved to be intimately linked to everything from obesity, diabetes, cancer, rheumatism and chronic bowel diseases to allergies and asthma.

This knowledge is already a basic element in the treatment of several of these chronic diseases. Some of the most popular medicines in the world have been developed to reduce chronic inflammation.

However, what few people know is that chronic inflammation has in recent years also been linked to many mental and neurological conditions such as anxiety, depression, bipolar disorders and perhaps even autism. There are also links to diseases such as MS, Parkinson's, the muscular disease ALS, cognitive impairment and Alzheimer's.

Not to mention the link to all of the preliminary stages and minor symptoms which many of us suffer from. This can involve everything from finding yourself staring into the fridge

49

without knowing what you're looking for to constantly catching minor colds and not having the energy to meet your friends and acquaintances.

Research within this area received a boost in 2015 when researchers discovered that the brain and the central nervous system have their own lymphatic system in which the inflammation could spread.

If a doctor takes blood samples from a mentally ill patient, it is very often possible to measure an internally smouldering inflammation. Unfortunately, such samples are very rarely taken.

Several years ago, researchers at Harvard University in the USA discovered that there is a link between Western food, chronic inflammation and depression. In 2013 they published the results, which were based on one of the world's very largest dietary studies: *The Nurses' Health Study*.

Their conclusion was that a diet of sugar, white flour, refined fats and red meat, especially processed meat, leads to chronic inflammation, and in turn increases the risk of depression.

In other words, exactly the kind of food that generations of us grew up with.

Of relevance here is the fact that the multiple Nobel prize-winning Harvard University has an extremely high reputation in the research world, and that several of the article's authors were among the institution's most respected authorities.

The same researchers could also demonstrate that a diet that contains better fats, lots of vegetables in general – and those high in fibre in particular – has an anti-inflammatory effect.

Several other studies in countries including the UK, Spain and Norway have also come to similar conclusions.

A basic rule for an anti-inflammatory diet is that fresh, healthy and little processed food is always better than old and highly refined. And ensure your diet is not too repetitive.

As we have already seen, whole grains are better than finely ground flour. But watch out for finely ground wholegrain flour! It's the size of the particles that's important. Meat from wild game and free-range animals is better than meat from animals reared quickly in crowded conditions. And you can add to this the fact that old, traditional plant varieties and animal breeds almost always result in more nutrient-dense foods than the new ones developed to produce maximum yields in terms of weight and volume in the cheapest possible way.

We think this is a really positive message. What's good for the animal and the environment is also best for our gut bacteria and our health – both physical and mental.

Suffering from the blood sugar blues?

You won't be surprised to hear that sugar and other refined carbohydrates with a high glycaemic index (GI) are among the most inflammatory things we can eat, but it bears repeating.

Normally, the amount of sugar (glucose) we have in the bloodstream is roughly equal to a sugar lump's worth. If we drink a 330 millilitre can of soft drink, which contains the equivalent of ten lumps of sugar, for the body it's like storing excess energy at lightning speed.

Blood sugar levels that are too high trigger inflammation and damage both blood vessels and internal organs.

To handle this surplus, insulin is secreted. This is a hormone that acts as a key to unlock fat cells so that blood sugar can enter and be stored there.

If we constantly feed ourselves with a lot of sugar or other carbohydrates that are quickly transformed into sugar in the body, the overfull fat cells eventually start to protest. The doors close and the

insulin key gets stuck. The cells are then described as insulin resistant, and the body's plan for maintaining uniform blood sugar levels doesn't work any more.

This is a precursor to Type 2 diabetes, a disease which has become one of the major conditions of our period. The seriousness of the situation is shown by a new estimate from China which shows that one in ten of the population is diabetic, and that one in two is suffering from the preliminary stages.

One of the biggest villains in this scenario is sweet soft drinks. It's hardly a coincidence that hot countries such as Jordan and Mexico are now leading the obesity league. And in Vietnam, more legs are now being amputated due to diabetes than as a result of mines during the Vietnam War.

Type 1 diabetes is caused by disruptions to the production of insulin,

51

and this disease is more genetic in origin, but even here scientists have recently seen interesting connections to the gut flora.

In many cases, "fast" carbohydrates and a reduced insulin response lead to the individual gaining weight. In the next stage, the full fat cells themselves begin to irritate the immune system. Obesity then becomes an engine that drives chronic inflammation.

This is the reason why fat stored inside the abdominal cavity is usually considered as being the most dangerous to health.

The abdominal fat is quite simply closer to vital organs to which the inflammation can jump (unlike bingo wings, for example).

When the doors to the fat cells are closed, the body desperately seeks another way to reduce the high blood sugar level. The solution it chooses is to store the excess in the liver.

This is a strategy that eliminates the acute crisis but can ultimately result in the life-threatening condition of fatty liver. This is a disease that is increasing rapidly, and which previously almost exclusively affected people with alcohol problems.

A popular solution that has been shown to be effective for many people in this situation is to eat a low-carb diet. Intermittent fasting – sometimes known as the 5:2 diet – can eventually lead to reduced insulin resistance and a more stable blood sugar level. When we don't eat carbohydrates, the body begins to produce its own glucose, which includes both the liver and fat cells emptying their stores.

But low-carb diets also risk backfiring by damaging the gut flora.

So a Western diet, for example consisting largely of pizza, white bread and soft drinks, may not merely make the blood sugar levels soar through the rapid uptake in the small intestine. Food that is free from fibre also starves out the friendly bacteria that live further down in the colon and which, from there, send out signals to regulate the blood sugar. We will look at how badly this can end on the next page.

The leaky gut

So we're back to chronic inflammation. What actually happens when it arises in the gut and ultimately makes us unhealthy? And how can we do something about it?

To answer this, we need to learn a little about what's known as leaky gut. It sounds disgusting! Perhaps not the most appetising subject in a cookery book. But we really must try to get through this section. Because it's *so* important.

One dramatic consequence when you have put your gut flora on a low fibre starvation diet is that survival instincts mean that normally peaceful bacteria in the colon start eating whatever is available – in other words you and your intestinal mucus!

It's like a hunger riot, with former friends turning against you – and on good grounds too, because you haven't looked after them properly. This contributes to what is known as leaky gut.

When the protective intestinal mucosa shrink, there's suddenly a chance for pathogenic bacteria to enter the microscopically thin intestinal wall (picture a sausage skin), which becomes inflamed and soon begins to allow penetration by unwelcome substances that can then escape into the bloodstream.

But as soon as you send down a new helping of fibre-rich food into the colon, your essentially well-disposed bacteria choose to eat that instead.

However, if the malicious bacteria are given free rein, that's the first step to a leaky gut. This takes place when the toxic substances present in the cell walls of these bacteria are released. These are called lipopolysaccharides, normally abbreviated to LPS.

The LPS toxin causes the mucous membrane to become inflamed and the very thin intestinal wall to start leaking.

If you imagine the cells in the intestinal walls as cobblestones, the narrow joints between them are passages where individual nutrient molecules from the food are absorbed.

In a leaky gut, these joints become wide and distended.

In normal cases, the intestinal wall only allows through the smallest broken down nutrient substances from the food. But now it suddenly allows the passage of larger particles which don't belong in the rest of the body but nevertheless jump on the train and out into the bloodstream.

Among the undesirable stowaways are the LPS toxin from gastroenteritis bacteria. In high doses, we develop gastroenteritis, of course, but even at low doses these bacteria can antagonise their surroundings and cause chronic inflammation. This is a new insight.

We can counteract a leaky gut both by eating less sugar and other carbohydrates that the body quickly converts to sugar, and by eating more fibre that nourish the gut flora.

Leaky gut has been linked with autoimmune diseases including rheumatism, cardiovascular diseases, neurological diseases such as MS and ALS, metabolic disorders including diabetes, with cancer and, of course, with mental illness.

Anti-inflammatory booster shot

So that we don't get too downhearted after reading this far, we probably need to perk ourselves up with an anti-inflammatory booster shot.

TOP TIP! 50 ml of this every morning is guaranteed to get your body and immune system going. We normally make one big batch a week and store it in the refrigerator.

serves 5–6

2 lemons
70 g ginger (about 7 cm of a
    thick-ish piece)
3 apples

1. Peel lemon and ginger.
2. Whizz everything up in a juicer
    (one with an auger).

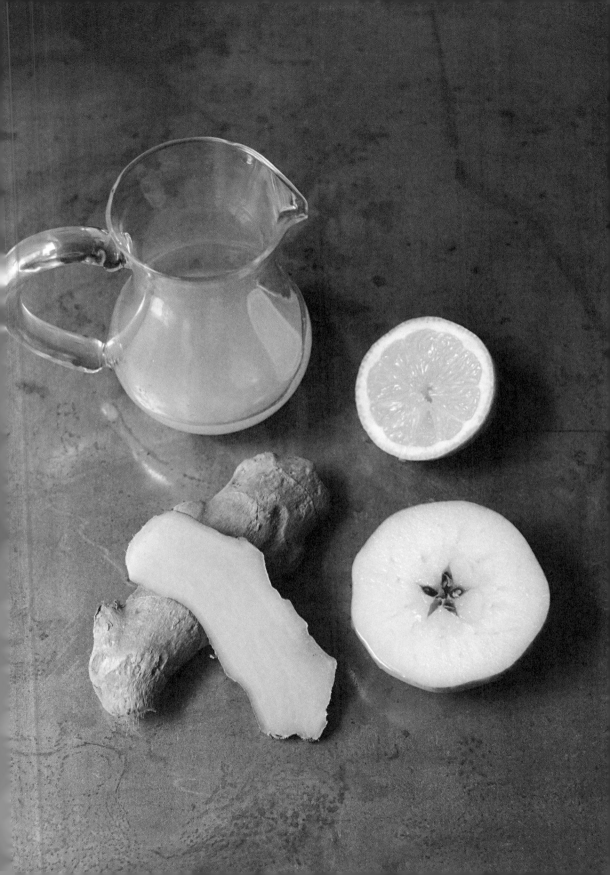

AGE and Alzheimer's

High blood sugar levels can lead to severe and even fatal damage to different organs, including the brain.

Raised blood sugar levels also cause something called glycation, where sugar and proteins bind together. This is roughly like when an old elastic band splits, except that here it involves your own tissue in the skin, blood vessels and heart valves. The substance formed is called AGE (see the glossary on the next page) and can easily be measured.

AGE increases throughout life and is usually reckoned as one of the most certain measurements of biological age.

I have tested my own AGE, which was a little below the result for my calendar age.

The first time was just after Christmas when I had been eating poorly for a little while, but I'm happy to say that you can improve your AGE value if you live healthily, which means that it might also be possible to rejuvenate yourself on a biological level.

AGE acts as a powerful prooxidant in the body. Oxidation is similar to when a car rusts, and it makes the immune system react by triggering inflammation. The link between chronic inflammation that arises as a result of high blood sugar and Alzheimer's is so strong that researchers have started to call the disease Type 3 diabetes.

By far the largest direct source of AGE from the diet comes from meat which is fried or grilled at high temperatures. Other sources are processed convenience food and pasteurised products, including hard cheese made from pasteurised milk.

In 2009, a study revealed that test subjects who ate a low AGE diet could reduce their values by a full 60% in four months. In other words, they became younger in biological terms. What did their low AGE diet consist of? As well as eating a lot of vegetables, they prepared their meat by poaching, steaming or using it in stews.

There's no particular reason to convert to eating only raw food for this reason. Because water is never hotter than 100 degrees, such cookery methods are sufficiently gentle and also contribute to facilitating the absorption of many nutrients.

AGE is also counteracted by vitamin E, which is found in foods including nuts and seeds. As we will see in a later chapter, there are many reasons to eat half a handful of nuts a day!

It's important to remember that pretty much all ingredients contain both healthy and harmful substances. We avoid some ingredients completely, such as fly agaric mushrooms. For others, the harmful substances can easily be removed by traditional cooking methods such as boiling and soaking.

Fruit is another example of an ingredient with both positive and negative substances. Although fruit contains fructose (if only in very small quantities), it also contains fibre and other substances with considerable health benefits. Even here, old varieties are preferable because the sweetness is often increased by intensive cultivation.

Many substances are also re-evaluated after a period, and where we have no absolute knowledge, a winning strategy is to rely on your own immune system and give it the best possible conditions in which to work. You do this by not overloading your body with a repetitive diet and by ensuring that it has a varied supply of vitamins, minerals, polyphenols and fibre. It's worth looking at how traditional healthy indigenous populations used to live.

GLOSSARY: sugar

Glucose: dextrose. Used as energy by muscle cells or stored in fat cells.
Fructose: fruit sugar. Not stored in muscle and fat cells, but instead goes directly to the liver where it is converted into glucose. The level in fruit is relatively low.
Blood sugar: glucose.
Ordinary table sugar: glucose + fructose.
Starch: how plants store energy. Consists of long chains of glucose.
HFCS: *high fructose corn syrup* is the cheap sugar from corn used in American soft drinks and sweets. It consists of around 55% fructose and 45% glucose. HFCS is not as common in Europe.
Glycogen: glucose when stored in the liver.
Insulin: the hormone that regulates blood sugar by placing the glucose in muscle and fat cells.
Insulin resistance: typical of Type 2 diabetes. Means that the cells no longer respond when the insulin wants to deliver glucose.
AGE: abbreviation of *advanced glycation end products*. This involves proteins reacting when they come into contact with sugar. AGE is considered to be one of several factors behind the ageing process and is considered to contribute to Alzheimer's.
Endotoxins: the toxins found in the cell walls of many gram-negative gastroenteritis bacteria. Also called LPSs, which stands for lipopolysaccharides. Are an important cause of chronic inflammation and probably also mental illness.
Leaky gut: when the thin intestinal wall becomes permeable to endotoxins and other harmful substances.

FOOD THAT CAUSES INFLAMMATION AND DEPRESSION

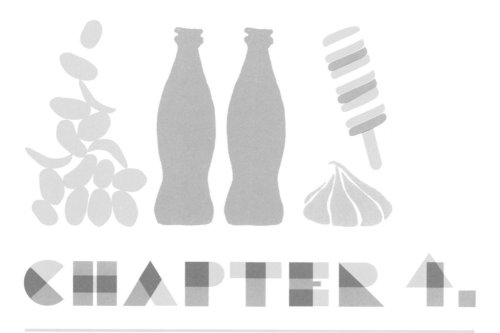

CHAPTER 4.

The happiness thieves in your pantry

To better understand what kind of food it is best to eat, we need to briefly draw your attention to the happiness thieves that it's sensible to clear out of your pantry.

Sugar

If you eat a lot of sugar, you have an increased risk of becoming depressed, and an increased probability of more aggressive development of diseases such as schizophrenia.

As we have already seen, sugar is deeply involved in the occurrence of chronic inflammation that affects both the body's various organs and the brain.

Countries with high sugar consumptions tend to have many cases of depression.

Of course, sugar also contributes to poor eating habits in general because it encourages us to eat junk food which is often full of sugar, bad fats and salt.

We used to believe that sugar primarily contributed to depression via increased obesity, which is a known risk factor for feeling down. But in 2017 two different research teams working on large studies for the first time reported a direct link between sugar and depression. According to one of these, the risk of depression increases markedly for anyone eating more than 60 grams of sugar a day. That's the equivalent of 20 sugar lumps. You can find this amount in half a litre of soft drink, or a breakfast consisting of a bowl of fruit yoghurt, sugar puffs and a glass of juice. 100 grams of pick-and-mix or a 100 gram bar of chocolate also puts you in the risk zone. And you can add to that the hidden sources in normal convenience food.

More than one in three Swedes eats more than 60 grams of added sugar every day. On average, we annually drink 100 litres of soft drink per person and eat 15 kilos of pick-and-mix.

Gluten and white flour

Finely ground white flour lacks fibre and is quickly broken down into sugars by enzymes in the small intestines. However, if the grain is eaten whole or coarsely cut it instead reaches the colon, where it becomes food for your bacteria. The difference in terms of health is enormous.

About 1% of us suffer from coeliac disease, a lifelong condition that means they can't tolerate the protein gluten, which is found in wheat, barley and rye. Other people too can be particularly sensitive.

One reason why intolerance to gluten and other fibre has increased is that our gut flora has been depleted and become unstable from a repetitive Western diet. The result is often inflammation, leading to both physical and mental disorders.

The gluten-free trend has brought benefits in that extremely one-sided overuse of finely ground wheat has been examined more closely. Many people have had their eyes opened to alternatives such as millet, the African seed teff and durra, which is a grass seed. But here too you need to be careful! Whole grain cereals are and remain a good source of fibre. If you stop eating whole grain cereals but don't replace this fibre with an equivalent, which isn't easy, your gut flora may be depleted.

Chemical additives

In 2014 researchers reported that sweeteners such as saccharin can disrupt the gut flora and cause obesity and Type 2 diabetes.

In the following year, worrying reports emerged that two E-marked emulsifiers – E 433 and E 466 – can damage the gut flora. In animal tests, they led to obesity, diabetes and the bowel disease IBS. Later tests on humans have confirmed that we are also affected in a similar way. Among other things, these additives resulted in significantly increased levels of a toxin that can be secreted by some gut bacteria.

E 433 – Polysorbate 80 is a stabiliser and emulsifier used in ice cream, sweets, chewing gum, soups, diet foods, and milk and cream-like products, for example in coffee machines.

E 466 – Carboxymethyl cellulose/ sodium carboxymethyl cellulose is a thickener and stabiliser used in ice cream, frozen chips and cheese.

These additives lead to a less varied gut flora and damage the intestinal mucosa so that inflammation occurs more easily. Such inflammation can be linked to depression.

Omega-6

The balance between polyunsaturated omega-3 and omega-6 fats is extremely important.

Omega-3 reduces inflammation and is found above all in oily fish, but also in a slightly less effective form in things like rapeseed and linseed oils. Omega-6 stimulates inflammation and is found in ingredients like corn and sunflower oils.

For millions of years, humans have eaten roughly the same amount of both of these variants of polyunsaturated fats, probably with some seasonal variations, as omega-3 fats are more common in nature in the spring and summer while omega-6 fats occur more in the autumn and winter. Today, omega-6 fats dominate throughout the year. The reason is primarily that the levels are high in corn and sunflower oil, which are often used as cheap fats by the food industry.

Pretty much all of us need to increase the quantity of omega-3 fats we consume and reduce omega-6.

What many of us don't know is that omega-6 is just a preliminary stage that must be converted in the body to the fatty acid (arachidonic acid) that is a direct cause of inflammation. Because not all omega-6 is converted, the primary source of arachidonic acid is actually meat, and above all chicken and other poultry. Fish and beef also contribute, but in smaller quantities.

Why is this? The answer is that the animal's own fat changes when it is given feed that contains a lot of omega-6. This also applies to eggs, which can be an excellent source of omega-3 if the chickens are allowed to range freely and peck at insects and larvae – but not otherwise.

- - - - - - - - - - - - - - - - - - - -

FACT: Flavonoids are a group of substances found in plants and which work as antioxidants.

- - - - - - - - - - - - - - - - - - - -

Refined fat

High quality, cold-pressed vegetable oils contain the full range of healthy flavonoids and oils. But when poorer quality fat is refined and processed, the results are unpleasant.

The most well known of these are trans fatty acids, which are produced when the unsaturated oils are saturated artificially so that they can be stored for longer on shelves without becoming rancid. Trans fats are fortunately becoming less common, but they are still present in our food. It is estimated that they lie behind millions of heart attacks – and are also linked to an increased risk of depression – since they were first introduced in the early 1900s as a way of preserving whale oil during long sea transports. They

61

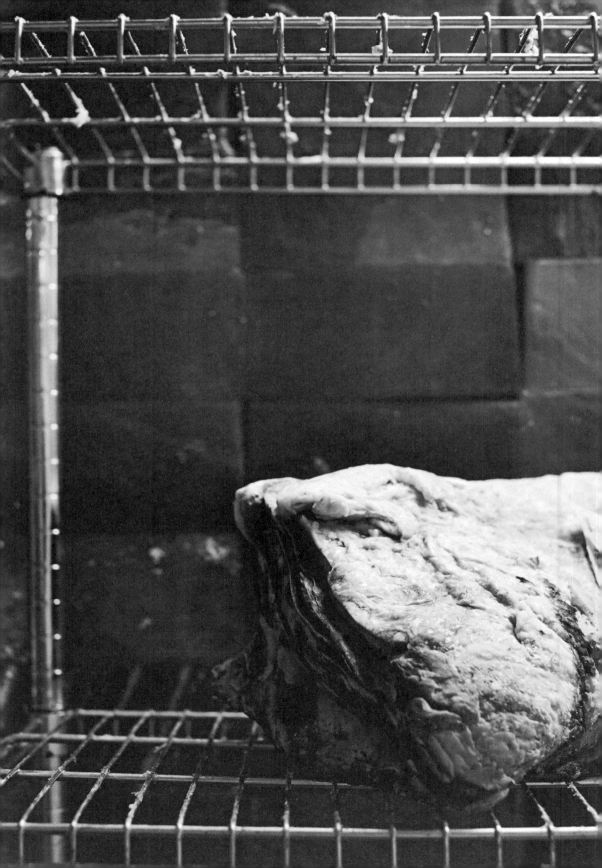

are a genuine killer, and yet they were awarded the Nobel Prize.

A reduction in the use of trans fats has opened the door for palm oil. The reason is that palm oil contains a lot of palmitic acid, a saturated fat which can also provide a long best-before date, but which has worse health effects than many other saturated fats such as stearic acid.

In addition to palm oil's highly publicised contribution to the destruction of the rainforests, it has recently been demonstrated that it forms hazardous substances which are carcinogenic or can damage the kidneys and testicles when it is industrially refined.

These chemical substances have also proved to cause inflammation.

Palm oil is a cornerstone in junk food and is found in almost half of all food products, not least cakes, margarines and convenience food. Avoid it!

Too much alcohol

A moderate intake of wine has been linked to the reduction of inflammation. "Moderate" means a glass of wine a day for women and two glasses for men.

Many studies show that there is a higher risk of depression among people who don't drink at all than among those who drink a lot.

Both the alcohol in itself and anti-inflammatory substances in the grape skins are thought to contribute to the protective effect of moderate drinking. The substance that has received the most attention is called resveratrol, which is found in the red colour in things like Concord grapes.

Moderate quantities of alcohol also seem to provide protection against heart disease, and here it's more the alcohol itself than whether you drink wine or beer. What's more important is how you drink and avoiding swallowing an entire week's worth at one sitting.

The question is controversial, because alcohol is also associated with an increased risk of many diseases including cancer. According to several studies, exercise seems to be an extremely decisive factor. In traditional cultures where people work hard physically and walk instead of driving, physical activity seems to neutralise the damage.

Of course the problem with alcohol is that many people find it difficult to drink moderately, significantly increasing the risk of disease. If you don't already drink, don't start! If you find it difficult to drink in moderation, stop completely!

The contents of wine don't have to be declared on the label, and wine can therefore contain additives that damage the gut flora. For this reason, natural wine is preferable.

HOW STRESS
AFFECTS YOUR GUT

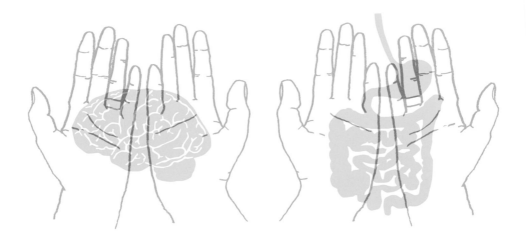

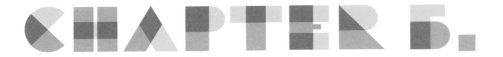
CHAPTER 5.

Stressed soldiers

We and our gut bacteria are actually very tolerant, which is why we may be able to handle some junk food. But this assumes that everything else is right, that we regularly get fresh air and take exercise. Or maybe if it was just stress, we could fix that too. But together, junk food and stress become more than we – and particularly our gut bacteria – can cope with. And if we start to tick off everything else in our environment and lifestyle, unfortunately there are often more things wrong than right.

Stress often seems to be the straw that breaks the camel's back. This was demonstrated in practice during a recent study of elite soldiers in the Norwegian Brigade Nord.

When they were exposed to extreme physical and mental stress during a four-day ski trek over open terrain, their gut leakage increased by 62%. The findings, which were reported in April 2017, constitute some of the clearest evidence thus far as to how stress contributes to chronic inflammation and increases the risk of other diseases.

It's common knowledge that if you're afraid and stressed your gut is badly affected, and that in the worst case you may even soil yourself. So it was hardly a coincidence that the military were interested in the link between stress and digestive health. In battle it's very important to have control of your emotions and not become paralysed by fear. The researchers' samples revealed that the stressed soldiers' faeces contained greater numbers of potentially harmful bacteria than normal.

At the same time there was a decrease in the levels of the bacteria that tend to dominate in a healthy gut – bacteria that can attack gastroenteritis bacteria, strengthen the immune system and work in an anti-inflammatory manner.

Have you ever thought about the fact that sometimes you get a stinking cold while at other times it seems like the cold virus just bounces off you? One explanation for this variation is stress.

There are other, earlier studies that suggest that the psychological stress of everyday life can be what ultimately causes the collapse of a non-harmonious gut flora.

Stress means that the immune system doesn't respond as well to the stress hormone cortisol. When the hormone calls a ceasefire, the immune system doesn't listen, but simply carries on, creating a great deal of unnecessary inflammation against imaginary enemies.

If we instead reduce stress levels, the immune system doesn't get stuck like this, and we feel healthier.

This failure of the immune system is considered to explain the relationship between external stress and the formation and progress of a whole range of diseases such as asthma, cardiovascular diseases, rheumatic diseases and mental illness.

In any case, the researchers who studied the Norwegian soldiers to understand how they could be most useful in battle came to a conclusion. Before the task begins, it is sensible to increase the number of stabilising bacteria in the gut. This could be done by serving the soldiers a range of alliums.

And from the outset, the soldiers could attempt to minimise the bacteria that increase under stress.

Guidelines prior to battle: eat onions, reduce fibre-poor junk food and eat less meat.

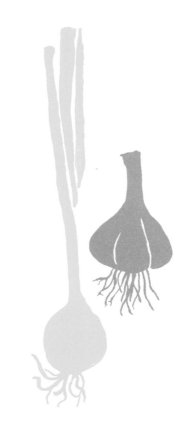

Rest your bacteria

Gut bacteria aren't merely sensitive to stress. They're also quite keen on following their daily routine, which includes a good night's sleep and food at set times.

In 2017 Swedish researchers reported that within just a couple of days, test subjects whose sleep rhythm was disrupted showed changes in their gut flora similar to those in people who eat junk food and become overweight.

At about the same time, Israeli researchers demonstrated that our gut bacteria follow an established daily schedule. In the morning they may produce a fatty acid, and then move onto manufacture hormones, changing later in the day to something different.

When they changed task they moved between different workstations in the gut.

It turned out that the liver – the body's waste treatment plant – was better able to clear toxins from the body in the morning than in the afternoon and that this related to the gut bacteria's daily schedule.

This research is still very new, but it's already clear that a stressful lifestyle with shift work, jet lag and food at irregular times can completely desynchronise our gut bacteria. And because the gut bacteria manufacture many of our hormones, this threatens to upset our own hormonal circadian rhythm so that we get even worse sleep problems and feel completely out of sorts.

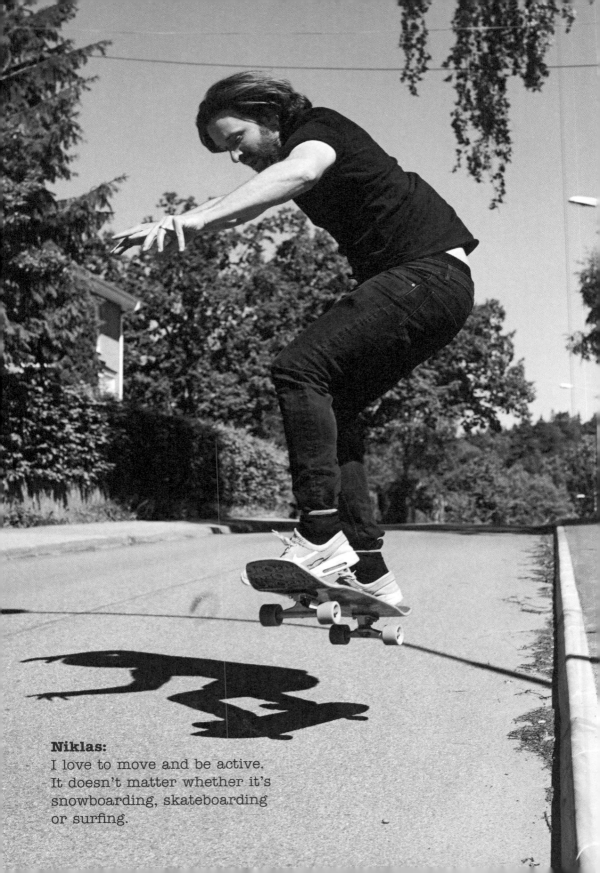

Niklas:
I love to move and be active. It doesn't matter whether it's snowboarding, skateboarding or surfing.

Exercise

For many years there has been very strong evidence that all forms of physical activity prevent depression. A major research review carried out in 2013 showed that the 30 best studies done in the field consistently indicated a clear preventive effect, even in less than 150 minutes of walking per week.

The mitigating effect has proved to be as good as that produced by the most common medications on the market.

The positive result works via a number of different mechanisms which are hormonal, blood sugar regulating and anti-inflammatory. The link to the gut flora is not as well explored, but in recent years results have emerged which demonstrate that exercise seems to have almost as strong an effect as food. For example, research has shown that exercise can almost completely prevent the negative effects on the gut flora that follow from eating junk food.

A study of rugby players also recently showed that elite sportspeople have a more varied gut flora than others. At the same time, extreme exercise can cause damage in the gut, so more research is required here to find the optimal level. But the general image produced by researchers is that exercise too can become an important future tool for achieving a healthy and stable gut flora.

FACT: New research shows that exercise increases the diversity of bacteria in the gut and particularly encourages the growth of friendly bacteria that help you feel better.

Happy Superfoods

[Anti-stress]

Chard: Stress can lead to depression, but it can be counteracted by chard! Leafy green vegetables such as spinach, nettles, dandelions, lettuce, endives – and why not ground elder? – are basic weapons in the anti-inflammatory kitchen arsenal. But chard may well be the very best.

The dark green leaves and the deep red colour of the stalks give away the rich content of vitamins such as A, C and B6, and not least magnesium which is often in short supply in people with depression. Chard is also extremely rich in antioxidants, including quercetin which is strongly anti-inflammatory and is being explored for its effect on cancer. Quercetin also counteracts a substance secreted in our brains when we are too stressed and which can make us depressed.

Celery: The happy food dark horse! Celery is rich in quercetin and kaempferol, which are thought to provide protection against depression caused by stress. Celery also contains the substance apigenin – a strong COX-2 inhibitor – which curbs inflammations as effectively as some medications. Apigenin is used in Chinese medicine for gout and rheumatism.

Celery also contains a number of substances that are being studied for their effect on both cancer and inflammation.

Celery is also a very good source of luteolin, which is one of few flavonoids that have been demonstrated to curb inflammation caused by allergens.

And you can add to this the fact that celery is a good source of vitamin K and potassium.

Omega-3: Recent studies point to omega-3 fat as one of the most active naturally occurring agents against depression.

In a traditional Mediterranean diet, people consumed sufficient omega-3 fat, in other words the fat found in fish, and in particular in the oily types such as salmon and mackerel. Herring is at least as good, and you only need quite a small amount every day to fulfil your requirements. Wild stocks of herring are also more stable than those of salmon.

Omega-3 has an anti-inflammatory effect and the body uses it in the most sensitive locations such as in contacts between the brain cells, in the eyes, sperm and in the heart valves. In a traditional Mediterranean diet, eggs from free-range hens and, to a certain extent, milk from freely grazing animals, also made a contribution.

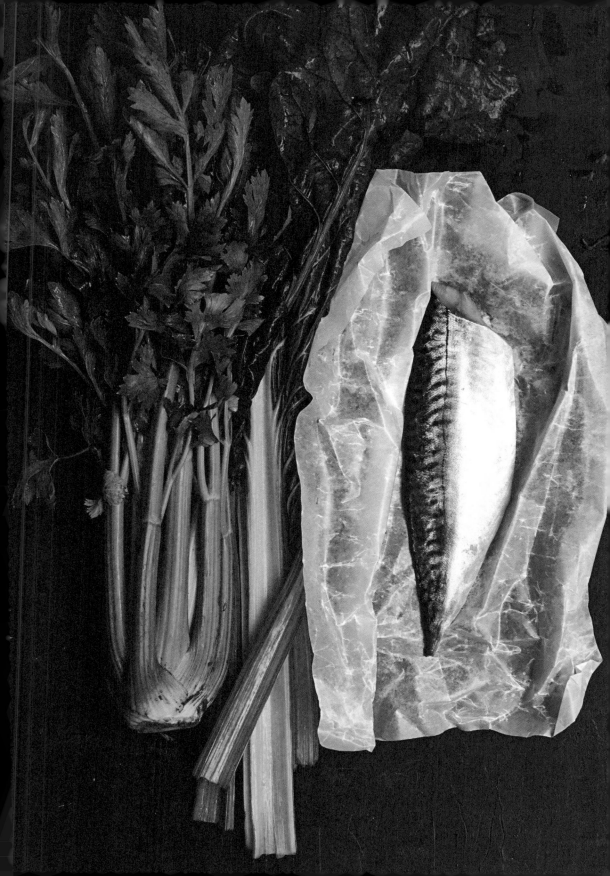

HOW CAN YOU EAT

YOURSELF HAPPY?

CHAPTER 6.

73 A warning about diets and detoxing. 74 Dietary advice for 2025.

A warning about diets and detoxing

There seem to be endless diets to choose from. But which one will make you happy? One American website lists more than 1,000 links to named books and members' clubs, and yet there are still other diets that I can't find here. There are always success stories about weight and health and almost all of them are based on excluding something from the diet. The evil thing must be removed. But this type of diet risks doing more harm than good.

Dieting in itself is a risk factor. In 2017 researchers reported that every time you go on a short-term diet by barely eating anything, you risk wiping out complete species of good gut bacteria, with the result that your modified gut bacteria make you gain weight even more quickly afterwards.

A bacterium lost can be lost for ever.

Other recent studies indicate that people who eat extreme diets that completely exclude different types of fibre also end up with depleted gut flora.

The risk zone contains those who completely avoid carbohydrates and those who don't eat enough fibre. Even gluten-free diets have been linked to an increased proportion of pathogenic bacteria in the gut. For those suffering from gluten intolerance, of course there's no other way, but the result shows how important it is to not prematurely exclude important types of fibre.

Should we also be careful about fasting? Here, there is thus far very little research about the effects on the gut flora, but given the positive health effects that result from different types of fasting, it's not something we want to caution you against. Particularly not if it involves short-term fasting (like the 5:2 diet), where the fasting periods aren't very long.

The consequences of longer periods of fasting and detox, and the point beyond which the gut flora may be affected, quite simply need to be investigated in more detail.

So now you know, there's no quick fix – you simply have to work out what type of foods your gut bacteria like. And we're going to look at that straight away!

Dietary advice for 2025

But does it have to be an effort? Isn't the good old plate model enough?

In July 2017 I was present during Almedalen Week, where I spoke about the series of articles on "Food and the psyche" that had been published earlier in the year in the newspaper *Svenska Dagbladet*. One unprepared question I was asked was: If you could change one thing in our eating habits on Monday, what would it be? In my brain – which right then was packed with new research findings – the answer was obvious: "A variation of fibre types that gives as wide a range of gut flora as possible!"

Amusingly, this response triggered a small Twitter storm among dieticians, who hadn't heard the entire conversation. One of them was the Swedish National Food Agency's director general, who liked and shared tweets saying that fruit and vegetables were perfectly sufficient and that the Swedish National Food Agency's dietary advice was more comprehensive.

My answer to these well-intentioned and committed tweeters is still that "fruit and vegetables" isn't sufficient guidance. No, the Swedish National Food Agency's dietary advice isn't more comprehensive. Different fruit and vegetables give us different fibres but in order to obtain a varied gut flora, we have to go further than that. And that is exactly what we must do, because an increasing proportion of the population expect to live longer than they might previously have done. This places new demands on what we eat.

The need for the type of deliberate variation in fibre types that we are talking about in *Happy Food* isn't something we have made up, but something that researchers around the world are in the process of discovering. This is something that will hopefully have left traces in the Swedish National Food Agency's dietary advice when it is revised in 2025. Sometimes even authorities can work quickly.

Yes, anyone who follows the dietary advice today has a good chance to have a more varied gut flora than someone eating junk food. We have many of the pieces, but in a random, unplanned manner. There is no analysis about how current dietary advice affects the gut flora. The dietary advice of the future must therefore include two things:

Variation in fibre types. A better definition of fibre, as the one currently used in the mandatory nutritional declarations on all packaged food products is so weakened that it's meaningless. Broad variation gives a broad, stable gut flora and lays the foundations for good health.

Nutrient density. We must rehabilitate the old plant varieties and breeding animals in order to be able to eat food that is dense in vitamins, minerals, good fats and polyphenols. They also taste and smell better into the bargain. Much depends on where in our long digestion apparatus carbohydrates are taken up.

The great thing about gut flora research is that it confirms every day that tasty, varied and well-prepared food that intuitively seems good for your health ... is good for your health.

Right at the beginning in the small intestine, or at the end when the food has reached the colon? It's the food absorbed in the latter part of the digestive system that can make you really happy, and we'll take a closer look at that in Part 2.

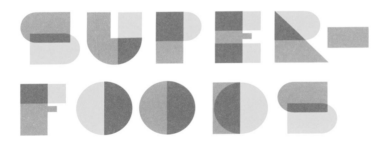

PRESENTING:
ING:

SUPER-
FOODS

Part 2.

In Part 1, we looked at the latest research into the link between unfriendly and friendly bacteria, the gut flora and our well-being. But what should we eat to be happy?

Part 2 is about the food. Join us as we explore the world's first proven anti-depression diet – a whole series of delicious superfoods, plus Niklas' recipes that work wonders for both body and soul. And best of all – you can change your gut flora in just 24 hours.

THE MEDITERRANEAN DIET THAT CREATES HARMONY

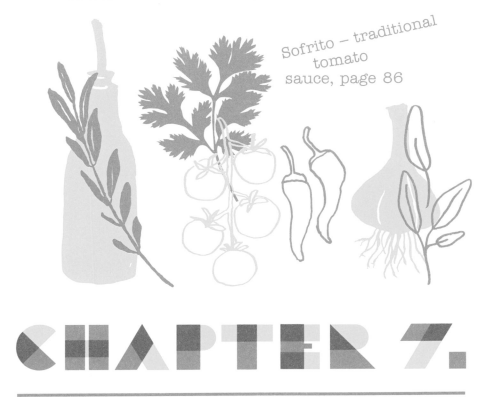

Sofrito – traditional tomato sauce, page 86

CHAPTER 7.

The world's first proven anti-depression diet

There's already a complete diet that's been shown to relieve depression – the Mediterranean diet.

So let's take a look at the World's First Proven Anti-depression Diet. This is the specially adapted Mediterranean diet that gave such good results against depression in the major Australian SMILES study in early 2017. Its formal name is the ModiMed diet, and it has more olive oil and nuts but slightly less meat than a normal Mediterranean diet. It was originally developed at La Trobe University in Melbourne.

No other oil has been as much studied as olive oil when it comes to the link with mental health. Normal food gives most people far more saturated fatty acids than recommendations advise. We're more likely to be lacking unsaturated fat, particularly omega-3, with the best source of this being fish. Many oils contain too much polyunsaturated omega-6 fat. One example which is better – or at least more neutral – than omega-6-rich sunflower or soya oils is rapeseed oil. It's important to choose cold-pressed oils and avoid refined vegetable oils where harmful substances are often formed during the manufacturing process.

Naturally, not everyone has to eat Mediterranean food to be healthy. Scandinavian food with a lot of fish and fresh vegetables and traditional Japanese food have both been associated with good mental health and well-being in major studies. But the strongest evidence so far applies to the Mediterranean diet, both from the above-mentioned Australian study where the ModiMed diet significantly reduced symptoms in roughly a third of patients with severe depression, and from another large study called PREDIMED. This began in 2003, and 7,447 Spaniards over 55 took part. This was an experimental study that also

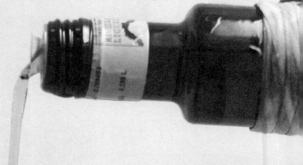

fulfilled what researchers usually call the "gold standard", but which was primarily designed to investigate the effect on the heart. "Gold standard" means that the test people are randomly selected, that it is a trial that can measure cause and effect, and that there is a control group.

The study is not only the largest ever of the Mediterranean diet, it is also the largest in the world to have examined whether it is possible to use food to prevent diseases in people who were originally healthy.

The results were presented on an ongoing basis, but the section relating to cardiac health was terminated prematurely in 2013 because the mortality rate was so much lower in the group eating the Mediterranean diet. It was simply not considered defensible to continue asking the control group to eat normal food.

Those eating the Mediterranean diet, which was reinforced with olive oil and nuts, reduced the risk of dying from heart and vascular diseases, including stroke, by one third.

This and other results have led to the Mediterranean diet today being the one that is proven to most surely lead to a reduced risk of dying prematurely.

A recent sub-study also shows that the Mediterranean diet is clearly more anti-inflammatory than a low-fat diet.

And, not least important for us, it reduces the risk of depression and makes us feel better!

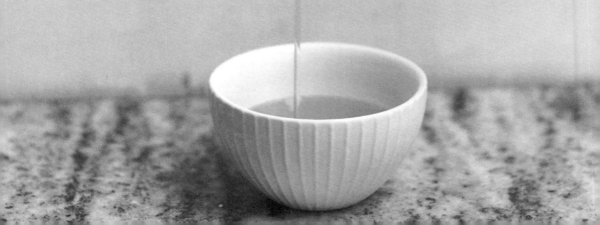

Anti-inflammatory olive oil and nuts

Many people are surprised when we say that the traditional Mediterranean diet is a high-fat diet. In the 1960s the Mediterranean diet was highlighted in one of the world's most famous dietary studies, the Seven Countries Study, which formed the basis of food authorities' long campaign for low-fat food.

If you think about it, it includes quite a lot of fatty foods, not least olive oil and nuts, but these are more unsaturated fatty acids.

The Greek island of Ikaria is usually reckoned to be the last outpost of the traditional Mediterranean diet. Here, fat constitutes almost 50% of the energy. Almost all of it comes from olive oil and the rest is lard.

Ikaria is a blue zone – in other words, one of the places on the earth where residents have the best chance to live to more than 100, and in good health. The people who live there live for almost ten years longer than the EU average.

I have visited the island several times, and when I'm there I think that I put plenty of olive oil on the salad, but still my local friends laugh at me, take the oil bottle and pour out twice the amount. Bread and salad bathe in oil, and I don't doubt for a second when they tell me that poor shepherds have many times taken a swig of energy-rich olive oil direct from the bottle for breakfast.

Yet despite this, the islanders don't get fat. The rest of the food is very low-fat, and full of herbs and different green vegetables.

Cold-pressed olive oil has long been pointed out as an important cause of the Mediterranean diet's healthy effect. But nobody could really explain why. Today we know that the olive oil contains several substances with anti-oxidative and anti-inflammatory effects, including quercetin, which is also found in blueberries and other healthy berries.

In 2005 an American researcher visited Europe. He had the unusual speciality of being an expert in medical scents. When he sampled the olive oil, he recognised a flavour that reminded him of the aftertaste of a painkiller.

It turned out to be a uniquely powerful molecule named oleocanthal, which functions in roughly the same way as best-selling NSAID painkillers like Ibuprofen and Ipren. Since then, various studies have demonstrated that oleocanthal can prevent both joint pain and Alzheimer's. In laboratory tests, it even has a strong inhibitory effect on cancer cells.

If you consume 50 millilitres of cold-pressed olive oil a day – which is still less than the normal average on Ikaria – this corresponds to one tenth of the recommended dose of painkillers. A low daily but lifelong intake might therefore be one of the secrets – but far from the only one – behind the Mediterranean diet.

However, you do need to use a genuine cold-pressed good quality virgin olive oil, and unfortunately there's a great deal of fraud in this area. You can recognise oleocanthal by the prickling taste at the back of the palate.

In the large-scale PREDIMED study, the Mediterranean diet's protective effect against depression was reinforced still further in those who ate a handful of nuts – around 30 grams – per day.

Nuts contain lots of fibre, including resistant starch. In general, they contain good fats and are full of minerals like magnesium and zinc, which many of us lack, and which are an important cause of depression and feeling off colour.

But obviously you have to avoid these if you are allergic, and you should also remember not to eat too many, as they provide lots of calories.

Fortunately, it seems that for some reason we actually don't go up in weight from eating nuts – in fact, rather the opposite.

In the largest survey thus far of public health on Earth, the *Global Burden of Disease*, financed by the Bill Gates Foundation, consuming too few nuts and seeds was the third cause of premature death and invalidity. In other words, millions of people on the planet die every year from eating too few nuts!

According to one of the other major diet studies, the *Nurses' Health Study*, you only need about a handful, ideally of varied types, in order to extend your life by two years.

The life-extending effect of eating nuts every day is the same as jogging for four hours per week!

Walnuts have been most studied and are usually associated with the biggest health effects, but the differences between different nuts isn't too great, and there's also a lot of research about hazelnuts and almonds. The most resistant starch is found in cashew nuts. Peanuts are also nutritious, despite actually being a legume rather than a nut. A personal favourite are Brazil nuts. And they don't merely taste good. One Brazilian study demonstrated that bad LDL cholesterol plummeted nine hours after the research subject ate four Brazil nuts! And, almost incredibly, the effect of these four nuts remained after 30 days.

One partial explanation can be that Brazil nuts are full of the mineral selenium, which many people in northern Europe lack because the soil is so poor in selenium. Selenium has an anti-inflammatory effect and is thought to counteract some forms of cancer.

Perhaps the research subjects had low selenium levels to start with. The biggest effects of supplements, in everything from vitamins to omega-3 fats, can almost always be seen in subjects with the worst starting point. Then the benefit of eating a little more tapers off very quickly.

One or two Brazil nuts a day covers your daily requirement for selenium. But to avoid something as rare as a selenium overdose, you shouldn't eat more than five Brazil nuts every day on average; 100 grams a month is ample.

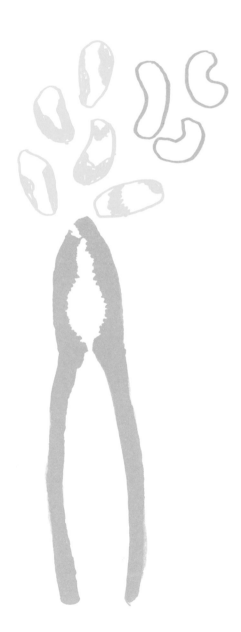

A quick guide

[To the Mediterranean diet]

1. The Mediterranean diet includes plenty of vegetables, fruit, legumes, whole grains, nuts, seeds, wild herbs and spices. It also incorporates lots of olive oil, dairy products in the form of cheese or yoghurt, together with fish and lean meat, often from chicken, sheep, goats or pigs, a few times a week.

2. The Mediterranean diet also includes drinking wine up to seven times a week – one or two glasses, and always with food. But note that this is traditionally entirely natural wine grown on their own land by people who work hard physically. In other words, this diet isn't entirely transferable to the way we live today.

The issue is controversial. Research in the Western world shows a slightly reduced risk of cardiovascular disease following moderate drinking, but an increased risk of cancer from relatively small amounts of alcohol. Overall, the risks outweigh the benefits. Interestingly, exercise even at relatively small levels seems to reduce, and in slightly larger quantities to completely neutralise, the risks of moderate alcohol intake. This was shown by a study carried out by Australian researchers published in autumn 2016.

3. The vegetables were grown on the subjects' own allotments without pesticides, sheep and goats were allowed to roam freely and graze, producing a good fat balance in both milk and meat, while the hens pecked at insects and laid eggs full of omega-3 fat.

4. The Mediterranean diet also has a positive effect on weight, waist measurement, osteoporosis, blood pressure, blood fats, inflammation, immune system, oxidative stress and atherosclerosis. Other results show that the anti-inflammatory effect is associated with longer and healthier telomeres, a known measurement of ageing.

5. Can we eat pasta or not? The answer for pasta is pretty much like for our potatoes: for traditional woodcutters who burned as much energy as top football players, it was fine to shovel in heaps of potatoes. The same applies to pasta for hard-working farmers and fishermen around the Mediterranean Sea. But anyone whose job is to tap on a keyboard all day burns far less energy. There's other food that's a better choice and which is richer in vitamins and minerals.

- - - - - - - - - - - - - - - - - - - -

In defence of pasta, it can be said that its dense texture means that the fibres reach slightly further into the gut than, for example, boiled potatoes. This makes it food for healing bacteria in the place where gut problems most often arise.

- - - - - - - - - - - - - - - - - - - -

Sofrito – traditional tomato sauce

Sofrito is the traditional tomato sauce used frequently in Spain, Portugal, Italy and also in Latin America. It's the Mediterranean diet version of French ratatouille. A super-tasty tomato sauce that can be used in all possible contexts and which is also packed with nutritious value.

serves 4

1 red chilli
2 red peppers
4–8 tomatoes
4 shallots, peeled
2 garlic cloves, peeled
3 tbsp olive oil
2 tbsp chopped parsley
    (or sage, basil)

1. Deseed the chilli and peppers.
2. Dice the peppers and tomatoes to roughly 1 cm cubes.
3. Finely chop the shallot, garlic and chilli.
4. Fry the shallot and chilli in olive oil over a high heat until soft but not brown.
5. Add the tomato and peppers and continue to fry gently for 2-4 minutes.
6. Top with chopped parsley.

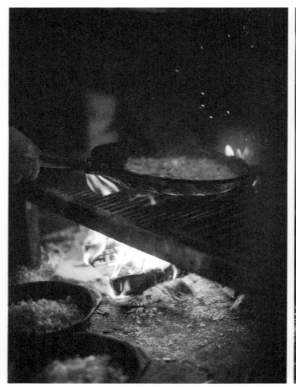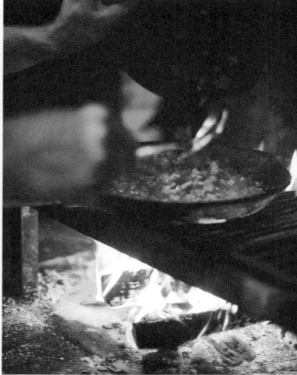

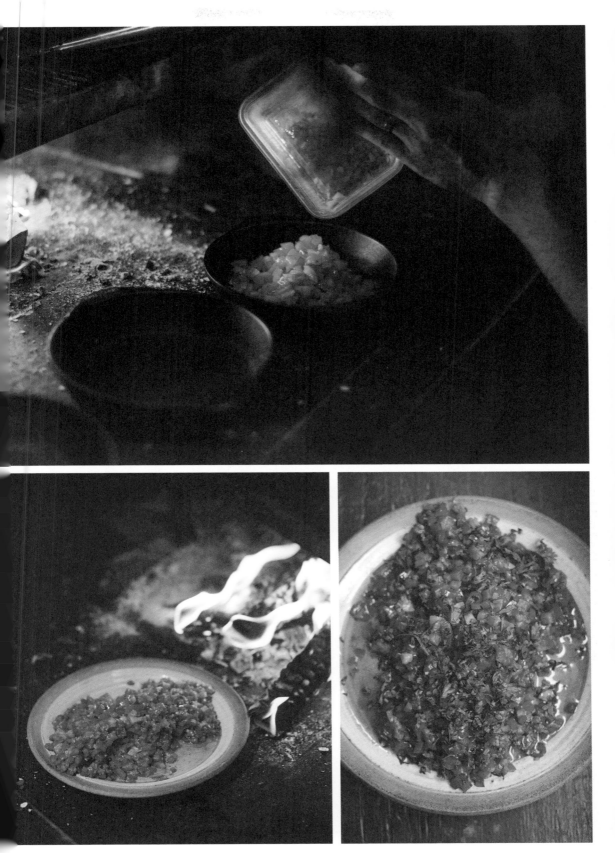

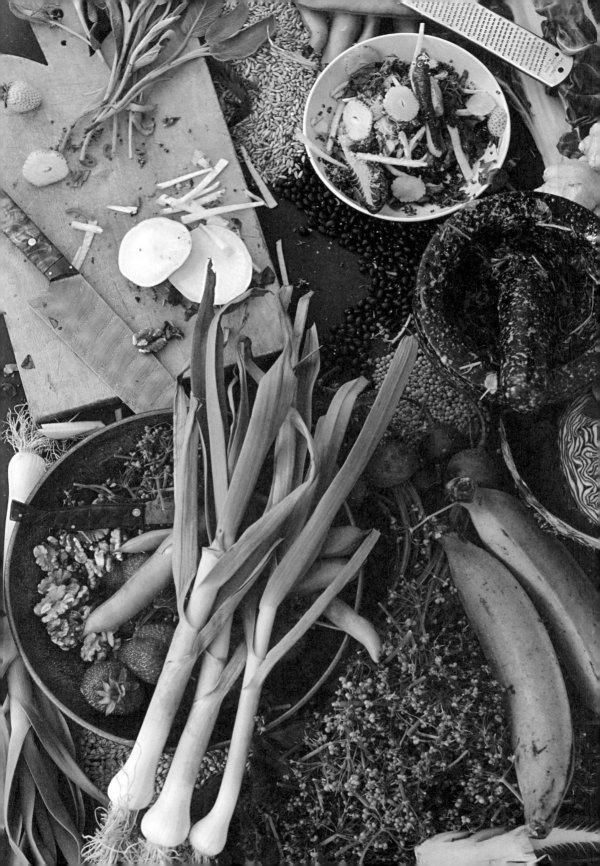

The anti-depression diet

[10 steps]

The Mediterranean diet that creates harmony

1. Eat vegetables at every meal – ideally leafy green vegetables and tomatoes every day.

2. Maximum one potato per day. Eat whole grains every day – the amount depends on how physically active you are.

3. Eat legumes 3–4 times a week, including in the form of hummus, for example.

4. Choose fruit, vegetables and nuts as snacks. Eat three fruit a day and 50 grams of unsalted nuts or seeds. 200 grams of olives are another option.

5. Eat oily fish at least twice a week. Eat eggs almost every day (maximum six per week).

6. Eat lean red meat 3–4 times a week – limit the amount to 65–100 grams per time.

7. Eat dairy products 2–3 times per day – for example feta cheese and natural yoghurt.

8. Use olive oil as your standard fat – roughly 60 milimetres of cold-pressed virgin olive oil every day.

9. Only eat sweet things in special cases.

10. Water is the best drink. Maximum 1–2 glasses of wine every day.

Happy Superfoods

[The good fats]

Olive oil: As we mentioned earlier, when combined with extra virgin olive oil, the Mediterranean diet relieves depression, according to a number of studies. One important reason for the positive effects of olive oil is the fact that it contains oleocanthal, which works in the same way as the best-selling painkiller Ibuprofen. Cold-pressed olive oil also contains a substance that neutralises the increased risk of atherosclerosis and heart attack in meat eaters. Balsamic vinegar and red wine in moderate quantities provide the same protection.

Other oils: If you prefer something other than olive, choose fresh and minimally processed fats such as cold-pressed rapeseed oil.

Cashew nuts: The Mediterranean diet reinforced with extra nuts such as walnuts, hazelnuts and almonds has been shown to be able to relieve depression. All nuts contain a lot of minerals and antioxidants and have an anti-inflammatory effect. However, the content of resistant starch varies. There is considerably more in cashew nuts and peanuts than in walnuts, Brazil nuts, pine nuts, almonds and macadamia nuts. But they all contribute different properties. About 50 grams of mixed nuts per day is a good dose.

Brazil nuts: Our personal feel-good favourite is still the Brazil nut. It's packed full of the three minerals that are most often in short supply in cases of anxiety and depression: selenium, magnesium and zinc. 100 grams contains almost 2,000% of your daily requirement of selenium, so you only need one or two nuts a day.

The main thing to remember is that we need a variety of fatty acids. Most people consume too much saturated fat and can therefore replace some of these saturated fats with vital polyunsaturated fatty acids. Fat from grass-fed or wild animals has a better fatty acid composition than from animals reared on concentrates.

Omega-3 fat in fish is linked to a positive impact on brain function. Rapeseed oil and linseed oil contain a precursor stage to these fatty acids, but they are not effectively transformed in the body.

We also need omega-6 fats, but we normally get these in excess via industrial fats based on soya, corn and sunflower oil. You can reduce these.

CHOOSE THE RIGHT OLIVE OIL

Olive oil is the world's most pirated product, either via pure fakes or diluted with cheap oils. Similar strategies can also be applied to other products such as good quality chocolate and coffee.

THE LABEL

The oil should be cold-pressed virgin olive oil, ideally certified by a third party. It is useful if the place of manufacture and not merely the country is stated on the label. The more exact this is, the better. The bottle should be dark and the date should state that it is a maximum of two years old.

THE PRICE

There's no guarantee that expensive equals good, although it's more probable.

AND ALSO

If you pay too little, you're undoubtedly getting a cheap oil.

IDEALLY

Get your own supplier. If possible, buy direct from the farm.

THE FLAVOUR

Tangy at the back of the palate, fruity and slightly bitter. Very little flavour indicates dilution, and olive oil should not taste of wine or be rancid. Carry out your own taste test with several different types, including bad ones.

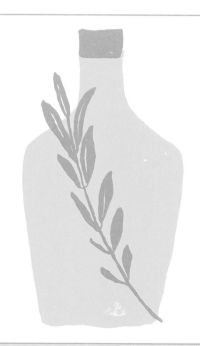

Cashew butter

A handful of nuts per day makes your body feel better.
All nuts are rich in fibre and minerals. Cashew nuts contain
a lot of resistant starch that nourish your good gut flora,
thereby contributing to many positive effects such as
balancing the blood sugar.

500 g cashew nuts
3 tbsp cold-pressed coconut oil
½ pinch salt

1. Cover the nuts with water and
    store chilled for 4–5 hours.
2. Strain off the water.
3. Mix the nuts, coconut oil and
    salt in a blender until smooth.
4. Store in an air-tight container
    in the fridge, where it will keep
    for several weeks.

- - - - - - - - - - - - - - - - - - - -

TOP TIP! Use cashew butter
as an alternative to butter
for spreading on crispbread,
for example. It's ideal for
use in raw food baking, but
also in normal cooking. We
use it as a filling in our raw
food bar on page 191. Try
it out with your morning
porridge, or, for increased
creaminess and flavour,
mix it into a smoothie
with berries.

- - - - - - - - - - - - - - - - - - - -

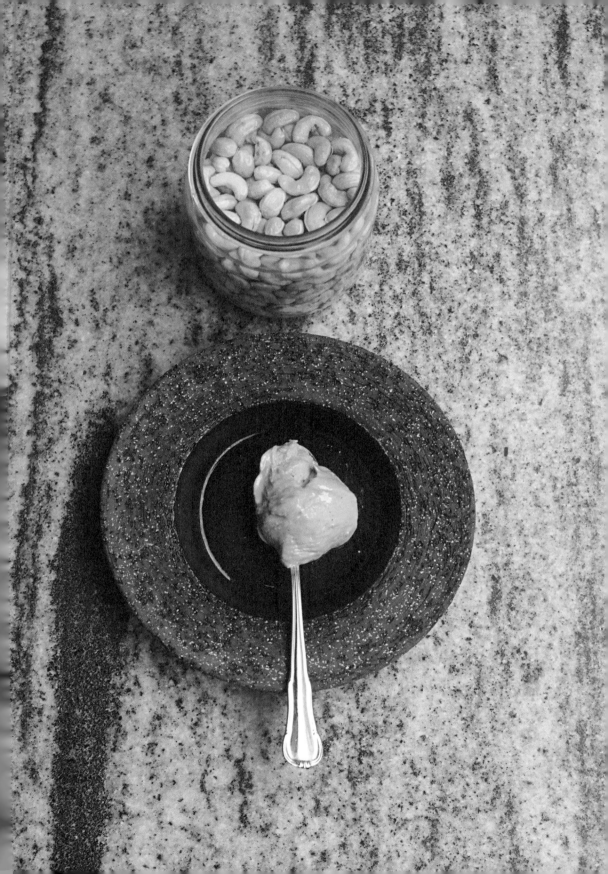

THE REVENGE OF
THE BEAN AND
POTATO GANG

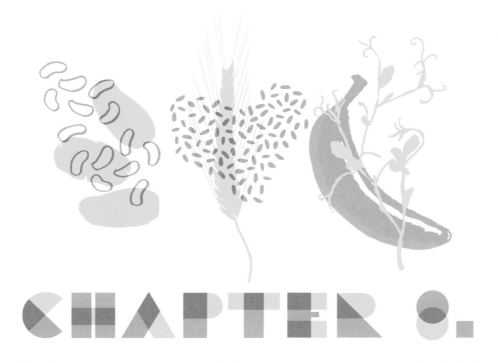

CHAPTER 8.

The bean diet

In spring 2017 I interviewed Patrik
Olsson, who lives in Halmstad in Sweden,
prior to the publication of his book *How
beans can change your life*. It is based
on his own tough experience of Type
1 diabetes, a disease that has made
him blind.

With 50 grams of beans immediately before and after each meal and a few intense strength training sessions a week, after 40 years Patrik Olsson was able to significantly reduce his insulin injections. He also lost 3.5 stone in two and a half months.

Patrik and his condition may be a special case, but Patrik's girlfriend also tried out the bean diet. She doesn't have diabetes, but suffers from insulin sensitivity, which means that she gains weight easily. When she added beans to her normal low-carb diet, she halved her weight, from 18.5 to 9.5 stone.

The beans also meant that, just as researchers had seen in their studies, her blood sugar curve fell significantly without her having changed her eating habits in other ways.

"It's amazing. I haven't stopped eating anything, simply added the beans. And my blood sugar has even reduced following meals," says Patrik.

Since Patrik described the bean diet in a Facebook group for diabetics, many others have tried it out and often reported extremely positive results.

Of course, nothing cures Type 1 diabetes, and those who suffer from this complex and largely genetically related disease, which can take many forms, shouldn't change their diet without talking to their doctor or dietician.

And yet from all directions we are receiving signals that beans and other legumes play a healing role in the gut flora and make us feel better.

The picture is the same regardless of whether we look at the eating habits of old people in the world's blue zones, where people live to be oldest and healthiest, or if we read international reports, interview cutting-edge researchers about their scientific trials or, as with Patrik, listen to the experiences of creative diabetics from their own kitchen experiments.

One explanation is undoubtedly that beans are a good source of what is known as resistant starch, but also that they contain other fibres.

Resistant starch

In early 2017 a research review was published that received attention from specialists all over the world. The reason was that, having re-examined many previous studies, the authors highlighted resistant starch as a particularly important component in anti-inflammatory food.

Why? Well, like other fibre, resistant starch is a form of carbohydrate that isn't broken down in the small intestine. But now it has been demonstrated that resistant starch doesn't just reach the colon but is also a master at attracting bacteria that produce short-chain fatty acids, and above all one called butyric acid. These fatty acids help the immune cells in the intestinal mucosa to proliferate.

The lack of such immune cells (called regulatory T cells) is considered to be a vital piece of the jigsaw that essentially links all "Western" diseases.

In other words, the more butyric acid formed and the healthier the gut with more T cells, the better you feel.

The most remarkable aspect is that we don't feed the gut ourselves – the bacteria do. But if you also remember that most chronic intestinal problems, including what's known as leaky gut, are closely associated with damaged intestinal mucosa, the benefits of getting resistant starch into place as quickly as possible become very clear.

In order to gain a serious understanding of resistant starch, we talked to researchers, including at the Karolinska Institute in Stockholm, and the University of Lund. They described to us how food is broken down in the gut. At the Food for Health Science Centre in Lund, for several years Inger Björck, Anne Nilsson and their colleagues have been studying how dietary fibre affects the gut flora.

To simplify a little, it's our own enzymes that do the majority of the work as the food first moves out of the stomach and through the small intestine.

The colon is where the bacteria take over. They can manufacture more than 3,000 different enzymes, which help us to absorb nutrients from the food. For example, while we ourselves can produce around ten enzymes that break down carbohydrates, our bacteria can produce ten times as many. So our own set of gut bacteria determines how sensitive we are to carbohydrates, and to everything else.

The colon is divided into three parts, and the problem is that almost all of the fibre-rich food we eat, and which gets that far, is dealt with by bacteria that thrive in the very first part of the colon.

This means that even if we eat fibre-rich ingredients such as Jerusalem artichokes, this only helps to create a healthy environment in the first part

FACT: Resistant starch
Starch is how plants store energy. The only thing that distinguishes it chemically from normal sugar is that the sugar molecules form long chains.

When these chains are a little shorter, they can be snipped off by the body's own enzymes, so that the pieces of sugar are ultimately small enough to be absorbed by the blood. This process begins in the mouth and continues in the small intestine.

The smaller these pieces of sugar are, the more quickly they are absorbed in the body. If we have poor blood sugar regulation and eat a lot of sweet things, we require a lot of insulin – the hormone that makes sure the level is correct – and then the blood sugar may instead fall too much, making us tired and lethargic.

This is what's normally known as the blood sugar blues. The worse your body handles blood sugar, the more your mood is likely to fluctuate. Sometimes rather hyper and sometimes sad and miserable. It's the same effect that makes you tired after eating.

So what's so great about resistant starch? Well, it has such long chains that they aren't broken down at all by our own enzymes in the small intestine. Instead, they become food for the bacteria living in the colon.

of the colon. But unfortunately almost all of the bad stuff that happens in the colon isn't there, but further down – often right at the end of the colon. The risk of a cancer growing at the end of the colon is 1,000 times greater than at the beginning.

In other words, this is where we want the food that can fertilise a friendly gut flora. Otherwise, the bad guys take over.

If we can succeed in this, the list of potential benefits is a long one. Very long.

The resistant starch contributes to reducing inflammation, but also to the production of hormones and signal substances which regulate the feeling of satiety and create a more stable blood sugar level. The latter is linked to the fact that butyric acid stimulates the production of a hormone called GLP-1 (why do all researchers love strange abbreviations?), which keeps the blood sugar constant. Healthier intestinal mucosa also reduce the risk of cancer in the colon.

This is good news for meat eaters, who otherwise run a greater risk, particularly if they aren't eating wild game or meat from free-range and grazing animals. If you really want to eat meat (and there are other reasons to hold back on this), add a few beans to your plate and neutralise the risk of cancer!

When Swedish researchers from a number of universities served a number of healthy research subjects an evening meal with normal, locally grown common beans (Phaseolus vulgaris), the positive effects lasted for 11–14 hours – in other words over several meals.

This is usually known as the "second meal" effect. This means, for example, that the blood sugar doesn't increase as much as normal at the next meal.

When the trial was repeated with whole barley grains, the effects were almost as striking. Whole barley grains also contain resistant starch. Just like when they ate beans, the test subjects' blood sugar levels were also lower during the following meals. At the same time, hormones that create feelings of hunger were inhibited, and blood samples showed that inflammation in the body had reduced.

Naturally, this is thought-provoking. In the West, beans and other legumes were basic foods just a few generations ago. Beans were the source of protein for the poor, but in line with increasing economic prosperity, beans have been overshadowed by meat, which hasn't exactly made our gut flora happy.

The same applies to barley. Before wheat took over, barley was the most common seed type, and barley porridge was one of the staple foods for most people, with a dab of freshly churned butter if they could get it. Like oats, barley also contains beta-glucans, a type of dietary fibre associated with good heart health and blood sugar balance.

Barley also contains a less well known fibre called arabinoxylan. It works as resistant starch, but in different parts of the colon. These two types of fibre complement each other extremely well and are an excellent example of how important it is to consume all possible types of fibre.

There are other types of fibre that can promote the production of butyric acid, such as inulin, which you can find in Jerusalem artichokes, garlic and other alliums, asparagus and chicory root, but none are as effective as resistant starch.

To encourage diversity in the gut, it's important to combine different types of ingredients containing different types of fibre. If you give Harry Kane all the attention but ignore the rest of the team, the game won't end well!

So how much resistant starch do we need?

To achieve the full effect for your health, the recommendation is that you consume 30 grams of resistant starch per day. Many traditional diets provide this amount, while in the Western world we eat much less – more like 7–8 grams per day.

Resistant starch occurs naturally in many foods, but specifically in legumes, linseeds and whole grains with the husk remaining.

And if, for some reason, you enjoy the harsh flavour of green bananas, these contain roughly 10 grams per 100 grams of banana.

That's twice as much resistant starch as ripe bananas.

Some brave souls have a teaspoon of potato starch in a glass of water in the mornings. This provides the pure substance. But it tastes a bit like wallpaper paste, so it's not our favourite snack.

If you're going to try to change your eating habits, it's much easier if the food is tasty and enjoyable.

Raw potato too – but not boiled – contains lots of resistant starch. In boiled potatoes that have been allowed to cool, some resistant starch reforms, so cold potato salad is a good choice. If you drizzle it with a little balsamic vinegar, even more is formed. Or why not fry traditional Swiss rösti made of grated raw potato?

Many people are worried about the carbohydrates in boiled potatoes, but despite being a slightly smaller proportion of the total, it appears that the resistant starch in cold potatoes can help neutralise the food's tendency to increase the blood sugar.

However, barley and beans are still the best sources of resistant starch.

Where can resistant starch be found?

There are three natural types:

1. Starch protected by a shell. Think of whole or coarsely chopped barley which will be protected on its way through the small intestine by its husk or size.

Found in: whole grains, lentils, bulgur, black or brown wholegrain rice, durra.

2. Starch of the amylose type which humans can't break down themselves with their enzymes.

Found in: raw potato, green unripe bananas, high amylose corn starch.

3. Resistant starch that reforms, for example if you allow boiled potatoes to cool. When the potato is boiled, the starch is broken down so that it can easily be absorbed in the body. When they cool, 10–15% of resistant starch is reformed.

Found in: cold potato salad, cold pasta and rice, cornflakes and similar. Tinned beans often contain higher levels than if you cook them yourself.

And one artificial type:

4. Modified starch. This is an artificial resistant starch which is often added to food products to provide structure. It is broken down to a very varied extent by the gut flora, so don't count on any positive health effects from this type.

RS shot

Potent shot of resistant starch

serves 4

4 tbsp potato flour
600 ml water
1 tbsp grated ginger
2 tbsp lemon juice

1. Blend all of the ingredients in a shaker or mixer.
2. Drink!

How much does your favourite ingredient contain?

There are almost as many measurement methods as researchers (why are they always so fussy?) but this is how much resistant starch is contained in around 100 grams of edible dry weight. The figure can vary slightly depending on the type and cooking method. There can also be other fibres in the same ingredient:

Barley (whole or coarsely chopped whole barley grain): up to 11–12 grams.

Oatflakes: 3–4 grams.

Lentils: 2 grams.

Common beans: 6.5 grams.

Other legumes such as chickpeas, black beans and kidney beans: 4–7 grams.

Green beans (boiled, cold): 6–7 grams.

Sweetcorn: 4.5 grams.

Corn tortilla: 3–4 grams.

Bananas: 1.3 grams.

Bananas (green): 8.5 grams.

Cooking bananas: 3–4 grams.

Cashew nuts: 12.9 grams.

Potato (boiled): 2.4 grams.

Potato (baked): 3.6 grams.

Cool boiled potato: 4.3 grams.

Potato (boiled, reheated): 3.5 grams.

Potato starch (unheated): 78 grams.

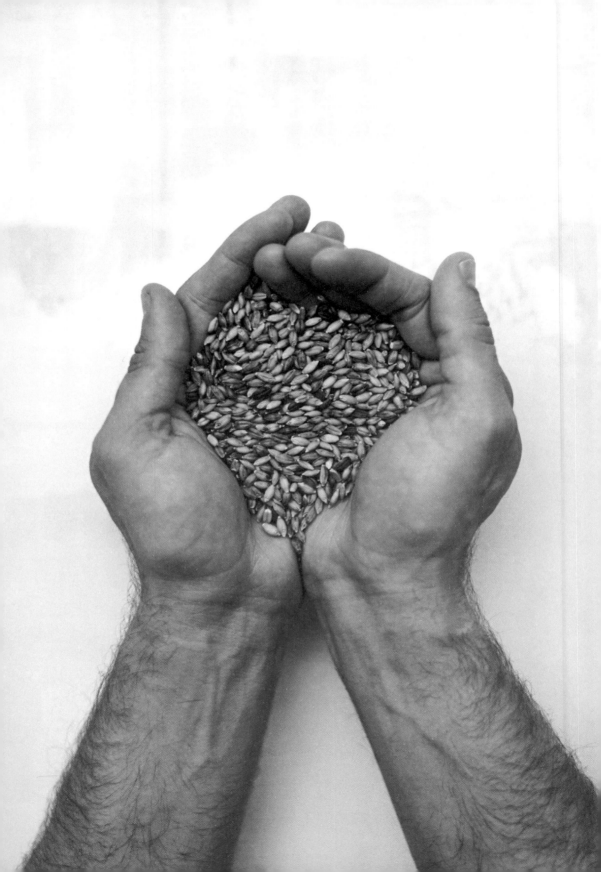

Happy Superfoods

[Beautiful beans]

Barley: Eat whole grain or coarsely chopped barley. Whole barley grains have emerged as one of the very best sources of resistant starch, in other words the form of starch that reaches furthest into the colon. Here it becomes food for bacteria that produce short-chain fatty acids. Butyric acid in particular has a long list of positive health effects, from helping the immune system and regulating the blood sugar to sealing the intestinal mucosa and preventing inflammatory toxins from penetrating the intestinal wall. In both traditional Mediterranean and Scandinavian diets, barley is a basic ingredient.

Common beans: All types of bean, with the possible exception of large white beans, are an excellent source of resistant starch. Traditional common beans (Phaseolus vulgaris) have been the best studied. Just like barley, they nourish the gut bacteria that produce the healthy butyric acid. The beans also balance the blood sugar so that you get what's known as a "second meal" effect in which the blood sugar is also kept stable for the following meal.

Chickpeas: People suffering from depression often lack vitamin B6, B12 and folate. Chickpeas are an excellent source of two of these – folate and vitamin B6. If you supplement these with liver, oysters or mussels, you also cover your requirement for B12.

Chickpeas also contain resistant starch, which helps the gut flora to produce butyric acid. A healthy gut flora manufactures its own B vitamins.

Barley porridge with blueberries and hazelnuts

Since the Viking period, people in the Nordic region have eaten barley porridge with a knob of freshly churned butter. Today we know that coarsely chopped barley is a good source of resistant starch and other healthy fibres. The substances in blueberries and other red berries and fruit help to keep your gut flora in shape.

serves 4

200 g barley groats
700–800 ml water
1 tsp salt
2 tbsp butter
100 g fresh or frozen blueberries
2 tbsp fresh honey
3 tbsp hazelnuts
200–400 ml milk (or plant-based
    milk such as almond or
    oat milk)

1. Place the barley groats, 500 ml water and salt into a saucepan.
2. Simmer carefully for 30 minutes, stirring occasionally, and dilute with more water to the desired consistency.
3. Top with a knob of butter, blueberries, honey, hazelnuts and milk.

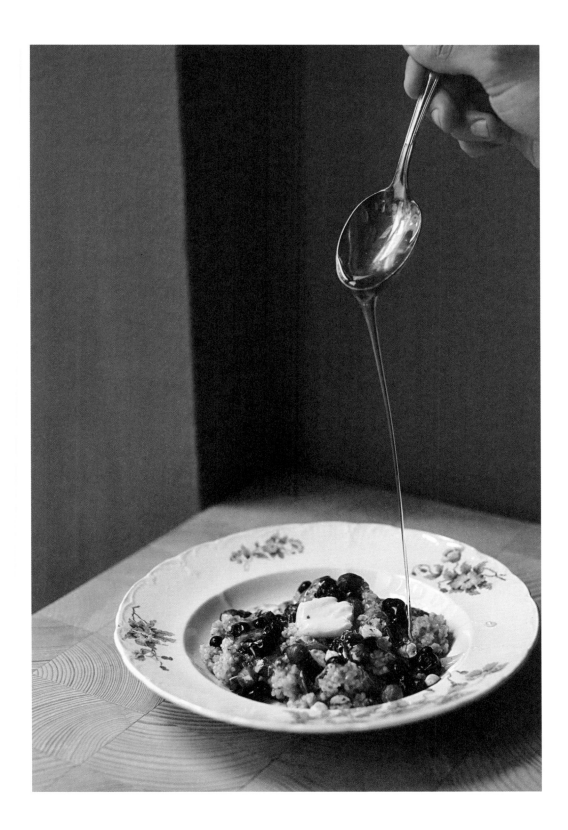

Mexican beans, black rice and corn tortilla

In Latin America, we have visited some of the places where people live to be oldest and healthiest. When we asked what they eat they all said the same thing: beans with rice and corn tortillas, every day, often for more than 100 years. Supplemented with a sea of colourful vegetables and a little protein. A winning concept that keeps both your taste buds and gut flora happy.

serves 4

1 yellow onion, peeled
2 garlic cloves, peeled
1 red chilli
3 cm ginger, peeled
1 tbsp olive oil
200 g dried black beans
2 tbsp tomato purée
2 limes, 1 freshly squeezed
200 g black rice
4–8 corn tortillas
1–2 tomatoes, sliced
6–8 sprigs coriander

1. Chop the onion, garlic and chilli. Grate the ginger.
2. Fry in olive oil over a medium heat while stirring for 2–3 minutes without browning.
3. Add the beans and tomato purée and continue to fry for 2 minutes.
4. Cover with water and allow to boil. Continue to simmer for 45–60 minutes, stirring occasionally. Add more water when required. The beans should be soft and cooked through.
5. Season with salt and freshly squeezed lime juice.
6. Cook the rice according to the instructions on the packaging.
7. Slice the lime and fry until golden brown.
8. Serve the beans with freshly fried tortilla, black rice, tomato, fresh coriander and fried lime.

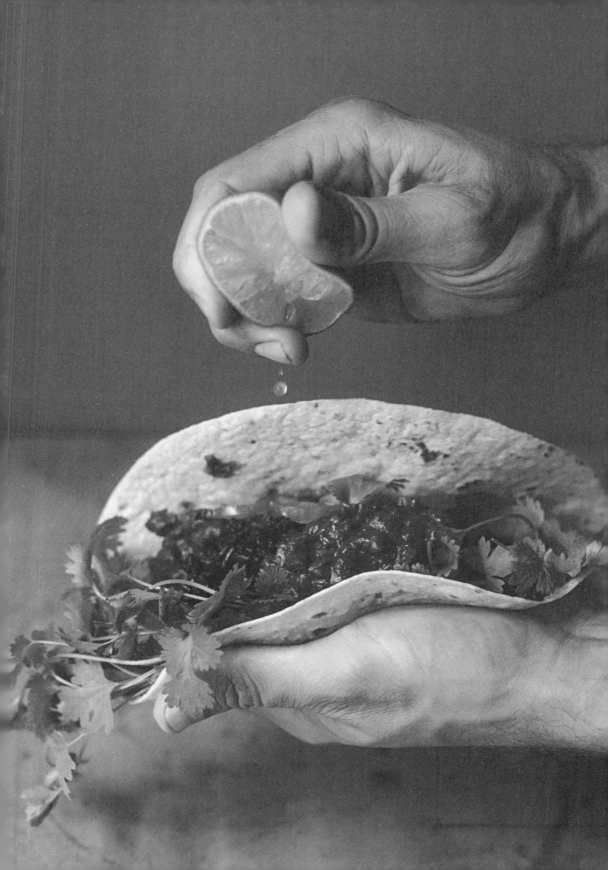

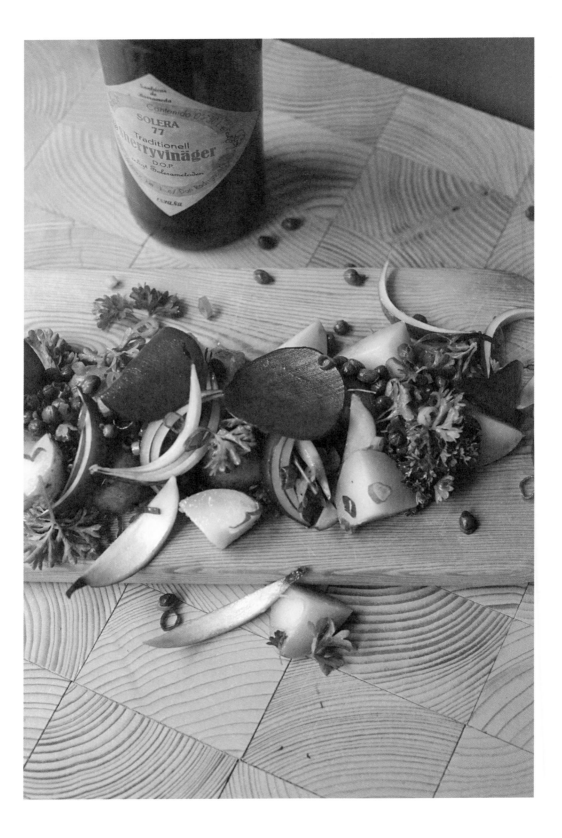

Potato salad with parsley, beetroot and vinegar

Potatoes have fallen out of favour for their high GI – in other words how much they raise the blood sugar level. But raw potatoes contain resistant starch which, on the contrary, contributes to stable blood sugar levels. In boiled potatoes which have been allowed to cool, some resistant starch reforms, and if you add a splash of vinegar there's even more.

serves 4

4–6 potatoes
1 red onion, peeled
2 tbsp red wine vinegar
3 tbsp olive oil
1–2 beetroot
1 bunch parsley, coarsely chopped
4 tbsp capers
sea salt

1. Boil the potatoes in salted water until soft.
2. Drain off the water, remove the lid so that the steam is released and allow to cool.
3. Cut into small pieces.
4. Halve the onion, then cut into wedges.
5. Mix the potatoes, onion, vinegar and olive oil.
6. Season with salt.
7. Slice the beetroot thinly over the potato salad, top with parsley and capers.

BRING IN
THE BEST FIBRE

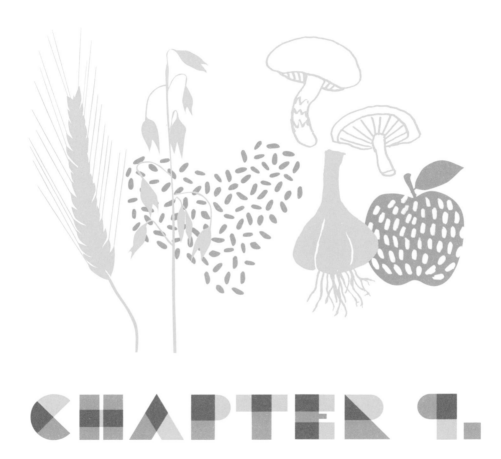

CHAPTER 9.

Finding your way in the fibre jungle

We've talked about resistant starch, which is found in beans and barley, and how it is good food for the healthy gut bacteria.

You really have to hunker down when the dietary winds are blowing! For years, carbohydrates have been discredited, but now they're coming back into focus on the side of the angels. And that's not as strange as it might sound. Around 100 years ago, British military doctor Robert McCarrison warned how processed food containing lots of sugar and very little plant fibre was causing epidemics of Western diseases in the British colonies.

McCarrison and other early pioneers realised that it wasn't carbohydrates in themselves that were a problem, but instead how they were processed, purified and over-consumed. According to them, the problem was both too much sugar and a lack of fibre. But at that point they knew very little about why fibre was good. Today we know more.

The fact is that there are hundreds of different variants of fibre. The secret is to eat many different types so that all of your gut bacteria are satisfied. If you want a varied gut flora, eat varied food!

Here are a few main groups that you should consume often:

Resistant starch: Best at forming butyric acid in the colon, even a little way in where the risk of inflammation is greater than in other areas. Found in things like beans, barley and other whole or coarsely chopped whole grains, in raw or cold boiled potato, lentils and green bananas.

Arabinoxylan: Good at producing butyric acid, particularly in the middle and final parts of the colon. Found in wholegrain cereal, especially barley, oats and wholegrain rice.

Inulin: Good at producing butyric acid, primarily in the first part of the colon. Found in vegetables such as asparagus and Jerusalem artichokes, and in onions, garlic and roots like salsify and chicory root. Primarily nourishes bifidobacteria, and together with FOS (see below) has produced weight reduction results in overweight children.

Fructooligosaccharides (FOS): Also known as oligofructan and sweet inulin as they have a sweet flavour. Found in fruit and in the same sources as inulin. Wheat and barley also contain FOS. Primarily nourishes healthy bifidobacteria, but doesn't produce as much butyric acid.

Beta-glucans: Good at creating butyric acid and regulating hunger and blood sugar. Found primarily in barley and oats but also in mushrooms and algae.

Pectin: Found to varying extents in fruit and berries. Higher levels in currants, lingonberries, raspberries, apples and citrus fruit. Highest levels in fruit that's unripe or only just ripe. Pectin is broken down in the freezer. Gives some supplementary butyric acid.

Wheat bran: The husk around the wheat grain isn't broken down in the gut, but counteracts constipation. Wheat bran increases the speed of flow in the gut and can help resistant starch and other fibre to reach further into the colon before being fermented into butyric acid.

Lignin: The only fibre which isn't a carbohydrate. Common in all plants. Not broken down in the gut. Just like wheat bran, good against constipation.

Chitin: Found in mushrooms and algae, in insects and the shells of shellfish. Can give traces of butyric acid.

There are hundreds of types of fibre. When we eat whole ingredients, we consume several types at the same time.

For example, if we eat Jerusalem artichokes, we consume both inulin and a lot of FOS. The FOS provides food for friendly bifidobacteria, while inulin can contribute butyric acid.

But when we eat semi-processed food with added fibre, there's a major risk that we will end up with an unhealthy preponderance in the gut.

Many companies that manufacture convenience food choose to use FOS and inulin because they have a sweet flavour. But in large quantities, added FOS and inulin can also cause growth of less healthy gastroenteritis bacteria. This can lead to stomach ache, gas formation and new imbalances in the gut.

It's hard to eat too much of natural ingredients such as Jerusalem artichokes, but the example demonstrates how important it is to eat a varied range of fibre that nourishes different types of bacteria. There's no point only eating resistant starch, nor inulin or any other type of fibre. You need a healthy mix of beans, whole grains, ideally boiled whole barley, onions, vegetables and fruit.

Then you and your gut bacteria will be happiest!

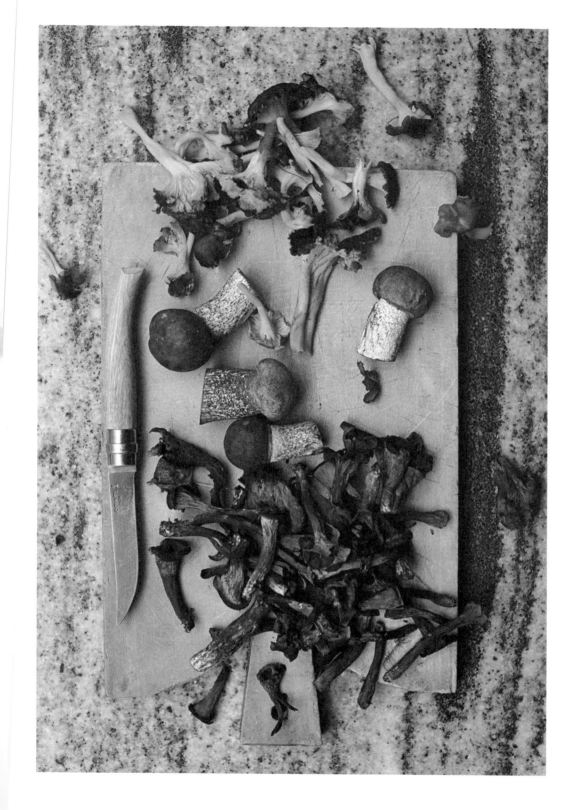

If you're not used to eating fibre, your stomach may start to rumble. It can take a while before the healthy bacteria grow, and it's a good idea to gradually increase the amount of fibre-rich food over several weeks. If you eat too much too quickly, you may even risk increasing pathogenic bacteria. If the symptoms don't go away, this may be something that doesn't suit your gut flora. Remember that we are all individual.

A significantly more common problem is that your gut begins to produce a lot of gas. This normally stabilises too, if you increase the fibre intake carefully. Fortunately it isn't dangerous, and in any case mainly consists of odourless gases such as hydrogen, carbon dioxide and methane.

Many of us – although not all – also have sulphur-producing bacteria in our gut. And you can tell this from the smell. These primarily live on vegetables that contain soluble fibre, like different types of cabbage. But there are also other sources that you may not be aware of, such as chewing gum containing sorbitol, the tap water in some places, meat and beer.

Those who are particularly fortunate can have a type of bacteria called Methanobrevibacter smithii, which lives from breaking down these types of gases. This means that you will break wind less than other people.

Unfortunately, almost all carbohydrates except for pure sugar

are now called "fibre". This has meant that the whole idea of fibre has been debased, which has contributed to food authorities being reluctant to allow health claims relating to fibre.

Many researchers have begun to avoid mentioning fibre and instead discuss MAC, which stands for microbiota accessible carbohydrates – in other words, carbohydrates that can be food for your gut bacteria. But not all fibre is appropriate for this. So the information about the quantity of fibre stated on food packaging doesn't say a great deal.

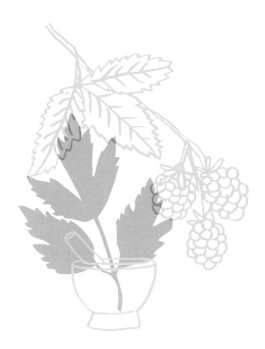

Fibre's route through the body

The mouth: The saliva contains the enzyme amylase, which begins the process of breaking down starch.

The stomach: Simpler carbohydrates (not dietary fibre) are split by various enzymes, producing simple sugars. The enzyme pepsin is also found here, which starts to break down the protein, together with hydrochloric acid that attack bacteria. Enzymes are like small scissors that trim the length of the molecules of protein, fat and carbohydrates until they're so short they can be absorbed by the body.

The small intestine: The short sugar chains are absorbed. On the way down from the stomach, gall and bile are added to the process. Gall works on fat so that it can be absorbed by the body, and also increases the pH value of the acidic gastric juice to facilitate nutrient absorption. The gastric juice also contains lots of other enzymes which break down proteins, fats and carbohydrates.

The colon: A reprocessing centre for anything left over. Food moves relatively quickly through the small intestine, but here the tempo slows and it can lie and ferment. Much dietary fibre is split by bacteria, which then increase in number. Some dietary fibre, such as wheat bran, cannot be broken down into sugars. This binds liquid and gives volume to the faeces.

Perfect poo

There are many theories about what form your poo should have to reflect a healthy gut flora. But, in fact, the transit time and volume are more important. This is to ensure uniform formation of butyric acid throughout the colon, but also so that hazardous substances don't sit in the same place in the gut for too long. If the food moves quickly through the colon, as it does during diarrhoea, the gut bacteria can't keep up. And if the process is too slow, we risk becoming constipated.

The dog food industry is expert in the matter of poo. Nobody wants to pick up sticky poo from the street, and you'd change dog food brand quite quickly if you had to do this often.

So the food is customised, which means that almost all dogs and cats are forced to live with permanent slight constipation, with poo that's dry and hard and with cracks in.

For us humans, there are two mechanisms that can mobilise a constipated gut. One is to eat quite large particles of insoluble fibre, such as wheat bran. This irritates the gut mucosa so that they secrete fluid.

The other mechanism is to eat soluble fibre such as psyllium (which comes from a close relative of the plantain). This binds fluid so that the stool becomes larger and more pliable, which means that it can more easily be massaged through the body by the constant movement of the gut.

Just don't forget to drink enough water so that the fibre can swell.

If you have a problem with poo that's too watery, the advice is also to consume soluble fibre, but this time with slightly less liquid. This works a bit like a sponge, absorbing the excess liquid. Where can you find soluble and insoluble fibre? In an apple, the skin is insoluble fibre, while the flesh is soluble. This is true for the majority of seeds, fruits and vegetables, and these are useful to counteract loose stools.

The weight is probably more important than the consistency. After 24 years' fieldwork in Uganda, one of the pioneers of fibre research, British children's doctor Dennis Burkitt, stated that a country where people produce small quantities of stools (poo) will need big hospitals.

In his most famous book, published in 1979, Burkitt describes how indigenous people in Africa often produce significant quantities – upwards of half a kilo a day. That's four times as much as many people in the Western world achieve. When the weight per day falls below 225 grams, the risk of colon cancer rises quickly. One tip is to weigh yourself before and after you go to the toilet...

So how long should the food take to go from your mouth to ... well, the other end? If you mainly eat a vegetarian diet, the passage usually takes one or two days. If you eat a Western diet that's free of fibre, it takes twice that long, or even more.

You can test yourself by eating beetroot and then keeping an eye on the colour. Around 36 hours should be considered an excellent time.

The colon has three sections, and they are normally emptied one at a time when you go to the toilet. In other words, your regular everyday routine can reflect what you ate several days previously.

A fast transit time and large volume are the objectives to bear in mind.

OK, so what's the perfect poo? Researchers can't quite agree about this. Some of them think that the normal consistency is relatively unimportant, provided that it's not small, hard bullets. Others recommend a shape that's more like pointy little mountains. Still others recommend the splash test: if you can easily produce a soft, long sausage shape without cracks that lands without a splash, you're doing well.

The best advice if you want to become king or queen of the loo is: eat wheat bran. Every gram of wheat bran produces 5 grams of solid poo. No other fibre comes close to it.

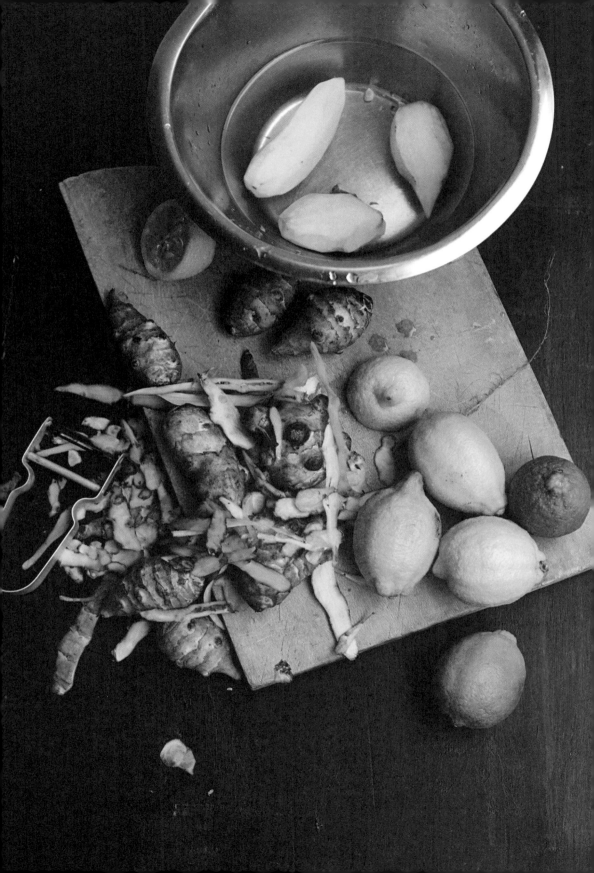

Happy Superfoods

[Fibre]

Jerusalem artichoke:
Contains the fibres inulin and fructooligosaccharides. When it is broken down by the gut bacteria, both bifidobacteria and healthy butyric acid are formed. Not as much as when you eat beans with resistant starch, but still a good amount. Inulin boosts the immune system, helps the gut flora and promotes the body's uptake of both calcium and magnesium. Inulin is often used as an added fibre in convenience food and also as a natural sweetener.

Garlic: Has been used for its medicinal properties since ancient times. Garlic contains a lot of the healthy fibre inulin. Various blogs also claim that garlic has a direct antidepressant effect, but there's not much scientific support for this. Generally nutritious? Yes. First choice for relieving mental illness? No.

Apple: All fruit contains pectin, which is one of the fibres that contribute to a richer gut flora and also to the production of short-chain fatty acids, including butyric acid. The proportion of pectin is actually highest in citrus fruit such as grapefruit, orange and lemon, but a lot of it is in the peel. One tip is to often grate citrus peel and use it in cooking because that's where so much of the nutritious benefits can be found. And make sure you avoid treated fruit, because traces of pesticides are often concentrated in the peel. Even berries such as lingonberries and currants contain lots of pectin.

Oats and rye: In both oats and rye we find several types of fibre which we recognise from barley. The difference is that the distribution is slightly different, with a slightly smaller proportion of resistant starch and slightly more beta-glucans and arabinoxylan, which also contribute to the production of butyric acid in the gut. Wholegrain rye has the highest fibre content overall of all cereals.

Tomato salad with whole rye and herbs

The increasing incidence of gluten intolerance has meant that many people have turned away from traditional cereals. But the effect is completely different when you eat seeds that have been ground into dust than if you eat them whole or coarsely crushed. Then they provide food for your friendly gut bacteria. Rye contains lots of healthy fibre, which your gut flora love.

serves 4

100 g whole rye
6–10 tomatoes, different colours
    and varieties
2 spring onions
2 tsp Dijon mustard
1 tbsp white wine vinegar
2 tbsp olive oil
1 bunch sage (or basil, dandelions,
    mustard greens)
sea salt

1. Cook the rye for about 40 minutes in salted water until soft.
2. Drain off the water, remove the lid so that the steam is released and allow to cool.
3. Cut the tomatoes into pieces.
4. Chop the spring onion.
5. Mix the tomato, onion, rye, Dijon mustard, vinegar and olive oil.
6. Season with salt.
7. Top with chopped sage.

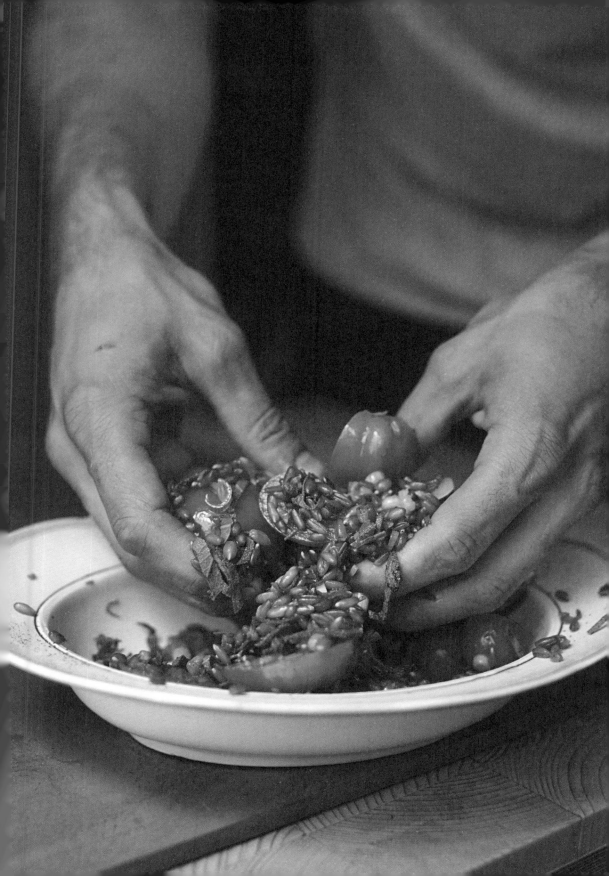

TOP UP WITH LIVING BACTERIAL CULTURES

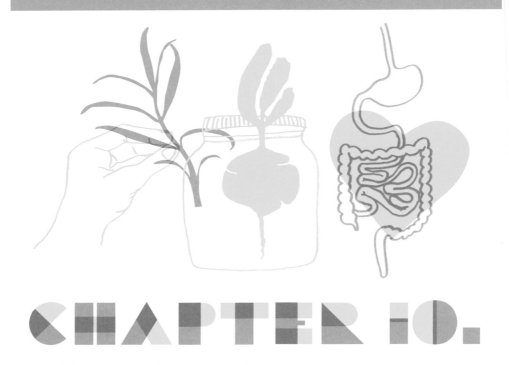

CHAPTER 10.

We all start as children

Food is the single most important way of looking after and developing a healthy, stable gut flora. But other things are also important, and several research groups are currently investigating whether the composition of the gut flora is established in the foetal stage.

At birth, a child's intestine is essentially sterile. The child receives the first dose of gut bacteria during birth, because the mother's vagina is usually, although not always, dominated by the same lactobacilli that you can find in live yoghurts.

In the case of Caesarean births, the first dose of bacteria that the newborn receives instead come from whatever happens to be in the birthing theatre.

This means that children born by Caesarean section often have a gut flora that contains fewer healthy bifidobacteria and more bacteria that are associated with worse health.

In many cases, of course, there is no safe alternative to a Caesarean section. But at the same time, it's important to remember that Caesarean sections increase the risk of the child developing an imbalanced gut flora. This can start with colic and end with a host of serious diseases – and even increased risk of autism.

According to one study, the increased risk of autism in the case of a Caesarean section is 22%, which corresponds to an increase from 10 to 12 cases per 1,000 births. In other words, a small risk increase in absolute terms. But there's also a clear link to a range of allergies and asthma, and to gluten intolerance and other digestive problems later in life.

So how worried should we be? We are still learning about this area, but clearly it should be taken seriously. A number of maternity wards have already introduced procedures so that children born by Caesarean section can lie adjacent to their mother's vagina for a while.

Another important factor in establishing the child's gut flora is breastfeeding. Here, too, knowledge is growing quickly and in 2017 a study was published demonstrating that around 30% of the child's gut flora is provided via the breast milk, with a further 10% from contact with the mother's skin during breastfeeding.

Other researchers have also recently demonstrated that fibre found in breast milk reduces stress and protects the gut.

The mother's breast milk is an excellent example of how totally dependent we and our gut bacteria are on each other. While the foetus is growing, the mother consumes about 300 extra calories per day. But to then produce breast milk, she consumes almost double – roughly 600 calories per day, indicating exactly how important the milk is.

The biggest energy consumption is a result of the mother manufacturing a form of very complex carbohydrate; fibres called oligosaccharides. There are almost 200 human oligosaccharides in breast milk.

The strange thing is that these can't be broken down by the child's own enzymes. So why do all mothers produce milk that the baby can't absorb?

The answer is that human oligosaccharides are excellent food for the friendly bacteria that the child needs in its gut.

In other words, mother's milk is largely made to feed the bacteria, not the child!

This is an example of how incredibly intertwined our lives are with those of our bacteria. This goes back to ancient times when life first appeared on Earth. Bacteria and other single cell organisms are so simply constructed that they often work together with other bacteria to gain access to abilities that they don't have themselves but need to survive.

An early dose of lactobacilli during birth and breastfeeding seem to create a breathing space for the child so that it can then build up a more varied gut flora. The early settlers multiply quickly and quite simply take up space so that the gut can't be invaded by yeast or gastroenteritis bacteria. This is an important period. Children who, from the age of four months are fed small amounts of cereal, for example, have a lower risk of becoming gluten intolerant.

Before the age of three, the child's gut flora stabilise in a way that is so individual that the gut flora has sometimes been compared to a fingerprint.

Another threat to the child's gut bacteria is overuse of antibiotics. Of course, antibiotics save many lives, but they should only be used when necessary. Listen to your doctor's advice. One reason is the risk of bacteria becoming resistant, but a standard course of antibiotics can also damage the gut flora.

The antibiotics don't distinguish between friend and enemy, and to reconstruct the gut flora following such treatment, probiotic capsules are sold in pharmacies. Normally, most bacteria recover, but there's a risk that some will disappear permanently and that your gut will be slightly more imbalanced for every course of antibiotics you take.

Interestingly, many mental and psychiatric problems first occur during an inflammation which has quite often also been treated with antibiotics. This is an observation that researchers around the world are trying to explore further.

Countless processes take place in the gut, and these can be sabotaged by antibiotics. In 2017 Danish researchers demonstrated that a single long-term course of antibiotics wipes out the inhibitory effect wholegrain rye can have on breast cancer.

Alongside antibiotics, modern humans have devoted a great deal of effort to eradicating bacteria. In our everyday lives we clean, take showers and wash like never before, and often using bleach, alcohol and other disinfectants.

It's hardly a coincidence that our gut flora has been depleted and allergies and asthma have increased at the same time that we have been waging war on bacteria. How intelligent is it to use antibacterial mouthwash when we know that a stable gut flora starts in the oral cavity? There are even studies showing that lactic acid bacteria counteract periodontitis and inflammation in the gums.

Lactic fermentation

As we have just seen, lactic acid bacteria are common in the gut of small children before they have established their adult gut flora, after which these bacteria are marginalised. They are stimulated by breastfeeding and physical contact with the mother.

But it is exactly this role as a vanguard that they also seem to be able to play in an adult whose gut flora has been disrupted. The bacteria break down simple sugars and transform them into acid, gas and alcohol. The most well known fermentation process is perhaps when yeast converts sugars into ethanol in beer and wine, but a more common end product in the gut is short-chain fatty acids such as butyric acid.

In any case, the lactic acid bacteria create an environment in the gut where other friendly bacteria can be happy and can grow in peace and quiet. This is a job they do well.

Lots of lactic acid bacteria can be found on normal vegetables. When the vegetables are allowed to ferment with these, this is usually called lactic fermentation.

The classic example is sauerkraut, but many vegetables can be fermented.

Human beings have fermented food for at least 8,000 years to extend its shelf life because the friendly bacteria become so numerous that they push out the bacteria that would otherwise make the vegetables rot.

Above all, lactic acid bacteria create an acid pH value where less friendly bacteria can't thrive. Into the bargain, the fermented food develops unique flavours that would not normally emerge.

But remember to watch out for ready-made fermented vegetables as these may only have been pickled in vinegar rather than fermented.

You also need to make sure that they have not been pasteurised. And that the product has been kept cold because otherwise you may be buying bacteria that are no longer alive.

We consume billions of bacteria with every meal. And yet the changes in our conservation habits, using refrigerators and freezers instead of fermenting food, have led to us now consuming far fewer and different bacteria than our ancestors.

You can also add to this the manufacturers' eagerness to sterilise food and add bactericidal preservatives to achieve a long shelf life.

We need to consume many bacteria because the majority don't survive all the way down into the colon.

The bacteria that don't perish in the acid bath of the stomach are corroded away by the bile in the small intestine. But a few of all those bacteria get all the way, perhaps because they belong to a particularly resistant family, such as lactobacillus rhamnosus and lactobacillus plantarum.

Others survive because they're hidden deep in a small piece of sauerkraut. You can also equip the bacteria with a protective film of fat, for example by mixing a little high-fat smetana into your live yoghurt.

Without doubt, reduced consumption of fermented foods is a contributory cause to the depletion of our gut flora.

A major review of research published in 2016 demonstrated that this type of living bacterial culture can reduce symptoms of anxiety and depression in otherwise healthy people going through stressful situations.

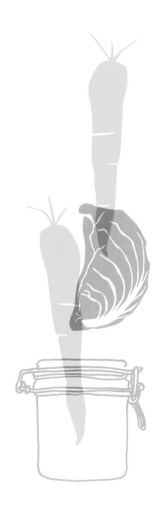

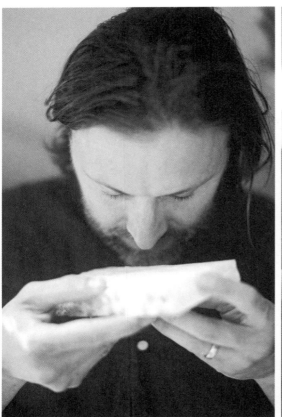

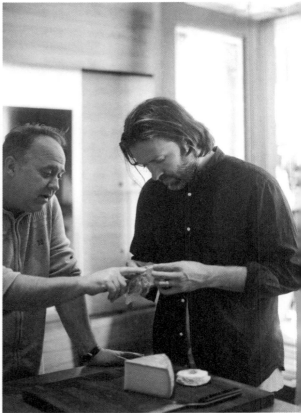

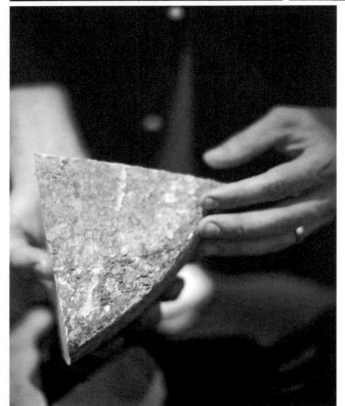

Unpasteurised cheese

Unpasteurised cheese contains broadly the same lactic acid bacteria as the expensive capsules you can buy in health food shops.

- - - - - - - - - - - - - -

TOP TIP! Serve as it is before dinner as an appetiser, as part of a salad or after dinner to extend the meal.

- - - - - - - - - - - - - -

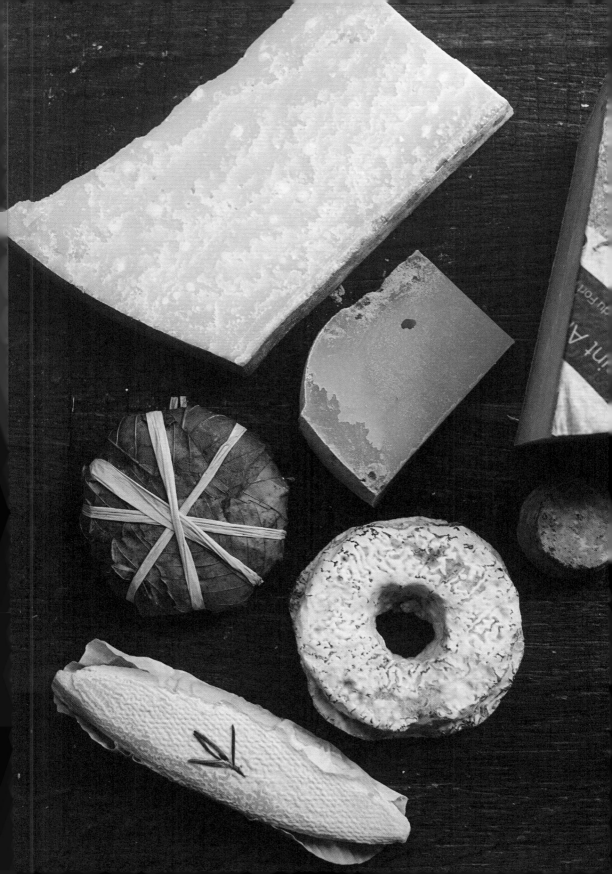

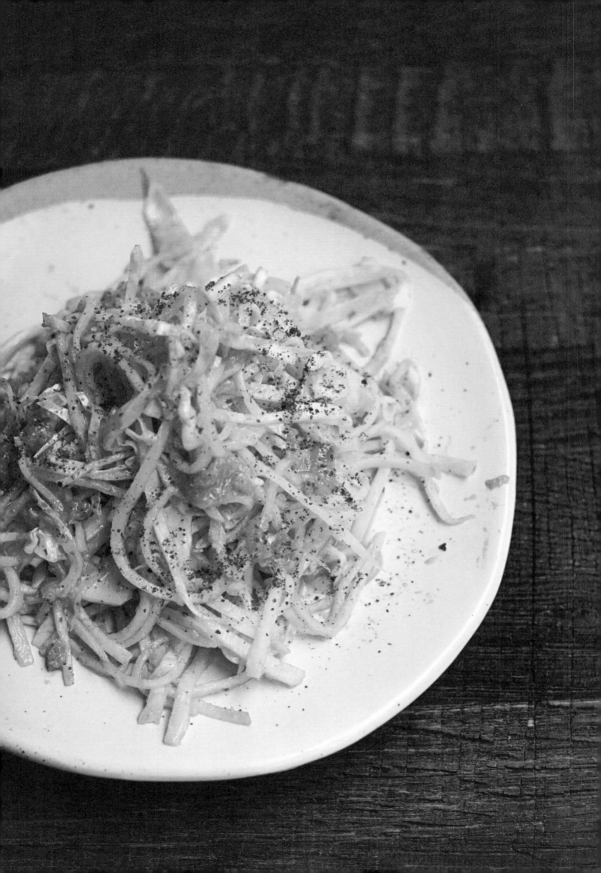

Kimchi salad

The Korean answer to sauerkraut is often based on Chinese leaf. Both kimchi and sauerkraut are vegetables fermented using lactic acid bacteria. Get into the habit of eating a little every day, but remember that this is a living ingredient which must be stored in a cold place.

serves 4

200 g ready-made kimchi
4–5 vegetables, e.g. courgettes, radish, green cabbage, carrots, spring onions

1. Mix the kimchi in a blender or with a stick blender until smooth.
2. Finely shred or thinly slice the vegetables.
3. Mix with the blended kimchi.

- - - - - - - - - - - - - - - - - - - -

TOP TIP! Fresh kimchi which hasn't yet developed a strong flavour is excellent as an accompaniment for many different dishes. In South Korea, it is often served with a rice dish called Bibimbap. When the kimchi has fermented for a couple of weeks, it will taste sharper and is ideal served with oily fish such as salmon and mackerel, or fried pork. Even more mature kimchi can be added to stir fries or stews.

- - - - - - - - - - - - - - - - - - - -

Sauerkraut

The majority of bacteria are friendly and help us to feel good. In the past – before the age of the refrigerator – people consumed far more bacteria than we currently do. Break the trend by choosing to eat a fermented product with living lactic acid cultures, such as sauerkraut, every day. Traditional Swedish isterband sausage is also fermented, although the bacteria die during the cooking process. But before this they produce a great deal of healthy vitamin K, which many people suffer from a lack of.

serves 4

1 kg white cabbage
1 tbsp salt without added iodine

1. Wash a screw-topped glass jar of approximately 1 litre.
2. Remove the outer leaves on the cabbage and discard.
3. Set aside one large white cabbage leaf.
4. Finely shred the rest using a food processor or thinly cut with a knife.
5. Place the cabbage in a large bowl and add 1 tbsp salt.
6. Knead the cabbage with both hands until it releases plenty of liquid.
7. Press the cabbage down into the jar, packing it in tightly, and leave a gap of a couple of centimetres below the lid, because the contents expand during fermentation.
8. Take the whole cabbage leaf and press down over the shredded cabbage so that it keeps the contents under the liquid.
9. Replace the lid.
10. Allow the sauerkraut to stand at room temperature for 7–10 days to start the fermentation process.
11. Open the lid once a day to release the air.
12. After 7–10 days at room temperature, place it in the refrigerator, where it will keep for months.
13. Perfect served with isterband sausage and French mustard.

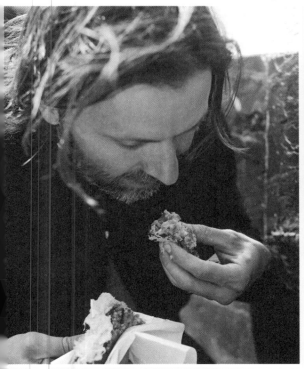

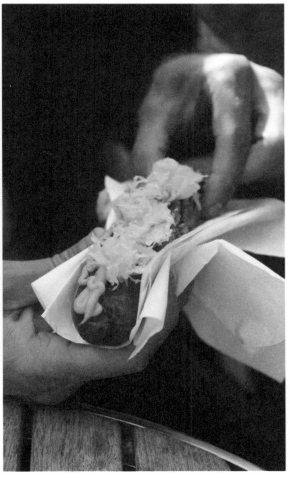

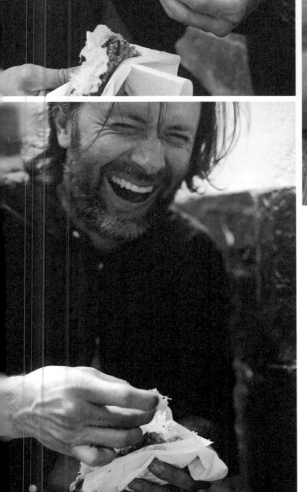

TOP TIP! How long you want to ferment it is entirely a question of personal taste. The jar can be left at room temperature for up to one month.

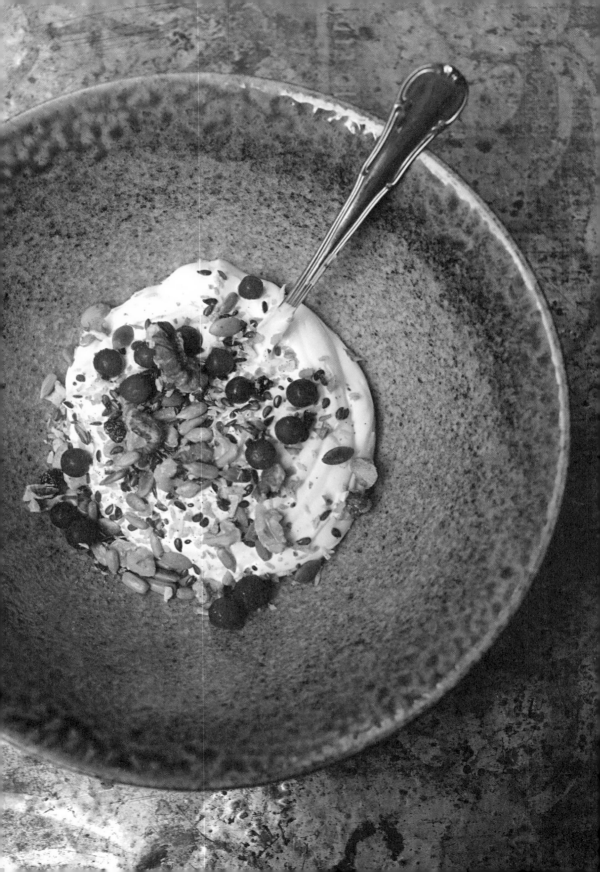

Kefir yoghurt

It's not difficult to make kefir yourself. You need kefir grains with a basic culture that you can buy online or in a health food shop. There are also groups on Facebook where people are happy to share.

Check the proportions for the kefir grains.

1. Pour room temperature milk into a clean glass jar. Ideally fresh, unpasteurised milk, but any milk will work.
2. Add the grains.
3. Cover with a tea towel held in place by an elastic band.
4. Allow the kefir to stand for 1-2 days until it has thickened. The time depends on how warm it is in the room and how many grains you use. If it's hotter than 30 degrees, the process is quicker.
5. Sieve the kefir and store in the fridge. You can now use the grains for the next batch.

Muesli

So simple, but so brilliant! The kefir contributes living lactic acid bacteria, but for them to thrive in the gut they have to get something to eat – such as muesli. It's a bit like sending your kids out with a lunchbox when they're going on a school trip!

serves 4

50 g mixed nuts
50 g linseeds
50 g sunflower seeds
50 g pumpkin seeds
50 g grated coconut
600–800 ml kefir yoghurt
50 g dried berries e.g. bilberries
    and cranberries
2 tsp ground cinnamon

1. Preheat the oven to 180°C without fan.
2. Chop the nuts coarsely.
3. Mix with seeds and coconut, and spread out on a baking tray.
4. Toast in the oven for approximately 8–10 minutes until lightly browned, stirring every other minute.
5. Remove from the oven and allow to cool.
6. Serve with kefir yoghurt, sprinkled with the dried berries and cinnamon.

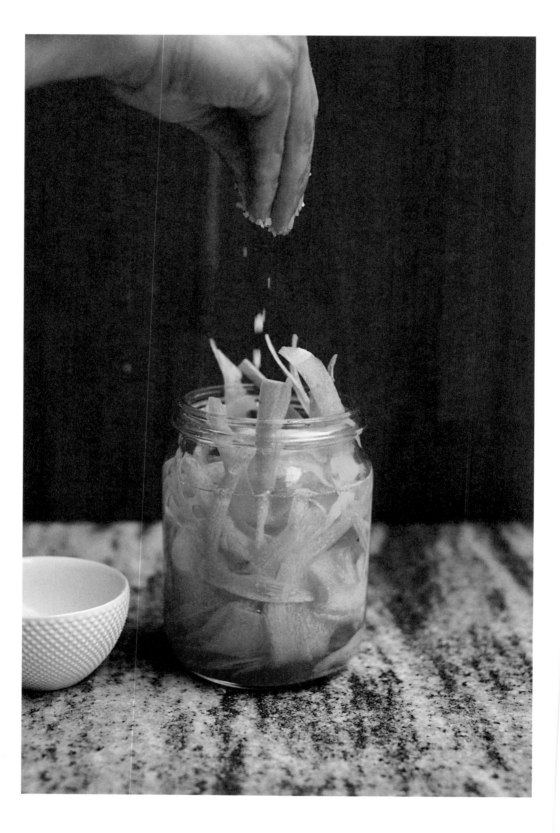

Lactic fermented vegetables

Start fermenting your own vegetables! It's easier than you might think. And tastier! Here's a simple guide to help you get started.

serves 4

½ kg carrots
2 tsp salt without added iodine
½ litre water

1. Wash a screw-topped glass jar of approximately 1 litre.
2. Peel and grate the carrots.
3. Whisk the salt in the water until dissolved.
4. Place the carrots in the jar, leaving a 2 cm gap at the top.
5. Cover with salted water.
6. Allow the jar to stand at room temperature with the lid on loosely for 3 days.
7. Screw the lid on tightly and place in a dark, cooler place, such as a cellar, for 1 week.
8. If you open the lid, it should smell fresh and acidic.
9. Close the lid and store in the refrigerator, ideally at the top where it isn't coldest, for 4–8 weeks.

- -

TOP TIP! You can replace the carrots with radishes, Chinese leaf, beetroot etc.

- -

Glossary

Probiotics give us new bacteria that make us feel healthier. These may be yoghurt or cheeses with living bacterial cultures, or expensive capsules. The problem is that they starve rapidly if they don't get something to eat. You have to consume a new helping every day.

Prebiotics are what you feed your bacteria. The majority of species are already in the gut, but there may be very few of them. If you nourish them, they increase in number. This is a more intelligent strategy than probiotics in the long run.

Synbiotics are when you do both things at the same time. You send down new bacteria and give them a lunch box. This is the health food industry's dream, and a great deal of research is done to develop expensive capsules. The alternative is to do it yourself.

Psychobiotics: The next step. Researchers hope that they will soon develop synbiotics that are tailored to making us feel good. But you can do the same thing at home in your kitchen.

On the hunt for bacteria

OK, we agree. It's a bit confusing to suddenly plan how we're going to consume MORE bacteria when all this time we've been hearing that bacteria are dangerous and that we should consume FEWER.

But even for Hippocrates, the father of medicine, who lived 2,000 years ago in Greece, it was clear that the way to good health started in the stomach. And bacteria are required in the stomach.

Towards the end of the 19th century, a Russian born professor named Ilya Mechnikov studied the long-lived mountain people of Bulgaria. He was convinced that their particularly good health was linked to their daily consumption of large quantities of yoghurt with live bacterial cultures.

The lactobacilli break down the milk sugar (lactose), which means that even lactose-intolerant people can usually eat this type of yoghurt.

But just when research into gut bacteria was about to take off, penicillin was discovered.

The triumph of antibiotics meant that bacteria as a group were largely forgotten. But in the wake of this came a hysteria for antiseptic cleanliness, in which everything had to be rubbed, scrubbed and kept clinically free of bacteria, ideally using a strong bactericidal product.

Even in Ilya Mechnikov's fermented milk products, all of the life-giving bacteria were now destroyed by heat during pasteurisation. This habit is now taken for granted, but it originally caused major protests and took decades for the large-scale dairy industry to enforce, against the will of small farm producers. Few things can make food authorities bristle quite as much as questioning pasteurisation of milk.

The concern is that people risk being infected with EHEC, which is an unpleasant, toxin-producing gastroenteritis bacteria.

139

There is a genuine risk, but the logical solution to the problem would be to clean up farms and stop the spread of EHEC among dairy cows.

A few years ago, there were suggestions in the EU to prohibit the sale of unpasteurised French cheeses. Fortunately, protests were so extensive that the idea came to nothing. Unpasteurised cheeses are therefore one of relatively few remaining natural food sources of probiotic gut bacteria.

Psychobiotics balance your emotions

Our gut flora don't merely affect our mental well-being and behaviour. John Cryan, who we met earlier, and his world-leading research group at the Microbiome Institute at the University of Cork in Ireland, have launched the theory that it is our gut bacteria that made us social creatures.

They and other scientists made this discovery when they realised that mice reared in a completely sterile environment, and therefore without gut bacteria, reacted differently to stress and demonstrated different social behaviour.

The researchers in Cork go so far as to say that our social ability is largely based on the fact that our gut bacteria benefit from us socialising with other people and therefore secrete hormones that make us open to new contacts. This makes it easier for the microbes to spread to new human hosts.

A normal mealtime means meeting other people. Handshakes, hugs and kisses on the cheek contribute to us developing a good, healthy gut flora in the colon. In other words it's not only the food on the plate that's important. The company around the table also contributes to pleasure on a much deeper level than we could have imagined.

For hundreds of thousands of years our ancestors have shared their gut flora with family and friends by eating from the same bowls and by physically living close to each other. We only began considering kisses on the mouth between friends as unhygienic 100 years ago – about when we started pasteurising milk.

In the past, family, friends and acquaintances must have acted as a collective reservoir for a common gut flora. An ecosystem that may have given rise to personalities with the same characteristics and dispositions.

In Denmark, *hygge* is the term for coming together over a good meal, lighting some candles and then sitting and talking for hours. Many people feel that this tradition is one of the reasons why the Danes are usually ranked as among the world's happiest people.

Meals have played the same central role in virtually all traditional cultures. But it's really only now that we are beginning to understand how many guests must really have been present at the table, when we include our gut bacteria.

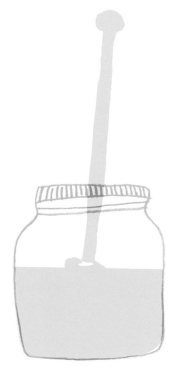

Happy Superfoods
[Friendly bacteria]

Sauerkraut: Lactic acid bacteria can be found everywhere in nature, and are transferred by both wind and insects. Those found naturally on a cabbage are sufficient to start a fermentation process if you follow a traditional recipe. After a little while, you have a product that contains 100 times more bacteria per gram than an expensive supplement and with a more varied flora into the bargain. The biological activity is so great that it's best to start carefully so that you don't give yourself digestive problems.

Many different food products are manufactured on the basis of this knowledge, including yoghurt, kefir, cheese, different sausages – and of course beer and wine.

You can find this type of food in many places in the world, for example in Korea with kimchi, which is often fermented Chinese leaf or ginger. In Asia fermented bean paste in the form of miso, tempeh and natto is common.

Often the same bacterial cultures, such as Lactobacillus acidofilus, are used in both expensive probiotic capsules and live yoghurt, and as starter cultures during lactic fermentation.

Honey: Ten years ago, Swedish researchers discovered that bees' own honey stomachs turn fresh honey into an extremely good source of lactic acid bacteria. With a full eleven types, including seven lactobacilli and four bifidobacteria, bee honey is the richest source of lactic acid bacteria so far discovered.

The living bacterial cultures mean that fresh honey has been shown to be able to overcome pathogenic and antibiotic-resistant bacteria. But after just a couple of weeks the bacteria have disappeared from the honey!

If you store fresh honey in the refrigerator or freezer, you extend the lifetime of the bacteria.

Honey was used as early as the Roman period to cheer people up. It contains a number of substances which have each been connected to better mental health. As well as tryptophan, which is the precursor to the happiness hormone serotonin, and which also contributes to good sleep, honey contains the healthy substances of kaempferol and quercetin. In research, both have been shown to have an antidepressant effect.

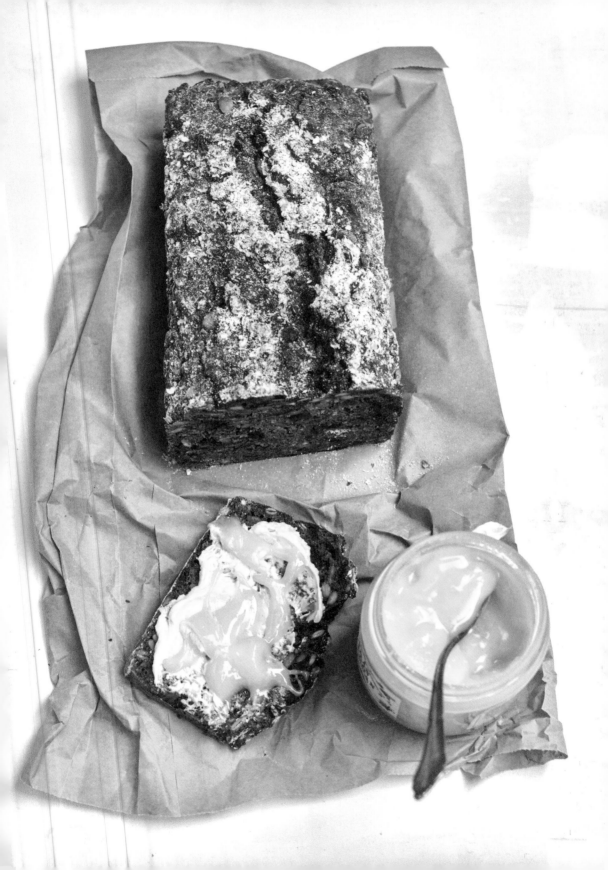

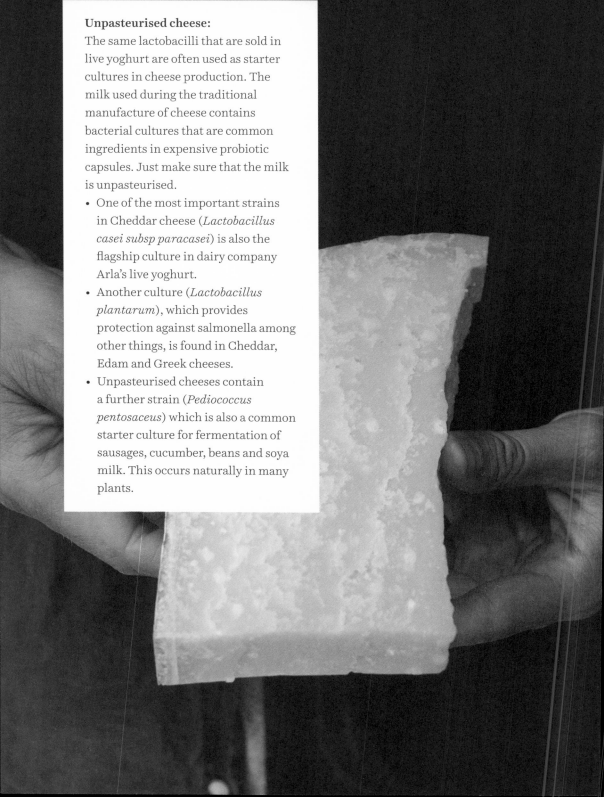

Unpasteurised cheese:
The same lactobacilli that are sold in live yoghurt are often used as starter cultures in cheese production. The milk used during the traditional manufacture of cheese contains bacterial cultures that are common ingredients in expensive probiotic capsules. Just make sure that the milk is unpasteurised.

- One of the most important strains in Cheddar cheese (*Lactobacillus casei subsp paracasei*) is also the flagship culture in dairy company Arla's live yoghurt.
- Another culture (*Lactobacillus plantarum*), which provides protection against salmonella among other things, is found in Cheddar, Edam and Greek cheeses.
- Unpasteurised cheeses contain a further strain (*Pediococcus pentosaceus*) which is also a common starter culture for fermentation of sausages, cucumber, beans and soya milk. This occurs naturally in many plants.

We raise a red flag

The internet is literally bursting with hyped probiotic products, but in many cases the scientific basis for these is fragile to say the least.

Unpasteurised vinegar: First the sugar in the grapes ferments so that alcohol is formed. In the next step, acetobacteria begin to convert the alcohol into acid. When all the alcohol has disappeared, vinegar has been formed. After this, the normal vinegar you buy is pasteurised. But unpasteurised vinegar, in which living cultures of acetobacteria can be found, has become very popular. Suddenly, unpasteurised vinegar is allegedly able to solve every possible health problem. But acetobacteria require oxygen to survive, and there's no oxygen in the gut. So these allegedly probiotic bacteria die very quickly and can't do any good at all.

However, the acid formed by the acetobacteria is antibacterial and has been used on cuts for several thousand years. Still, consuming large amounts of vinegar is of dubious benefit. If you reduce the acid content of the gut too much, you risk not only wiping out gastroenteritis bacteria, but also damaging the friendly bacteria.

One of the advantages of vinegar is that it helps to increase the proportion of resistant starch in other food, such as cold potato salad. There are other advantages of vinegar: better blood sugar regulation, better heart health, better nutrient uptake and preferential formation of things like vitamin K, but this has nothing to do with living bacterial cultures.

Pasteurised balsamic vinegar works just as well.

Kombucha: Here is another major trend that you shouldn't be taken in by: fermented tea. The kombucha hype originates in Hong Kong, and here too there is no good research that demonstrates if and how the living culture affects the health. In kombucha, the mother culture consists largely of yeast, an area in which we have significantly less knowledge than in the case of gut bacteria. Nor are the bacteria thriving in kombucha among the most prominent in the human gut flora.

Of course there are many people who say they feel good because they drink kombucha, but this is currently more a matter of belief than of scientific evidence.

Steamed vegetables, pumpkin seeds and olive oil with sea salt

This is a dish inspired by the evening meal of steamed leaf vegetables often eaten by the inhabitants of the Greek island of Ikaria. This island is one of the blue zones where people live longest while remaining healthiest. Steaming is a gentle method for preserving the plants' healthy polyphenols.

serves 4

3 tbsp pumpkin seeds
½ butternut squash
1–2 heads of broccoli
1 green cabbage
3 tbsp olive oil
1 tbsp sea salt

TOP TIP! Can also be cooked in lightly salted water, but remember to halve the cooking time.

1. Place the pumpkin seeds in a frying pan over high heat. Toast while stirring for 2–3 minutes until they have browned.
2. Pour out onto a large plate to cool.
3. Peel the squash and use a spoon to scoop out the seeds.
4. Slice the squash into 1 cm thick slices.
5. Peel the stalk of the broccoli and cut the rest into florets.
6. Remove the leaves from the green cabbage.
7. Set up a steamer.
8. Start by steaming the squash for 2–3 minutes, then add the broccoli and cabbage. Continue to steam for 2–4 minutes.
9. Place in a bowl and serve with olive oil, pumpkin seeds and sea salt.

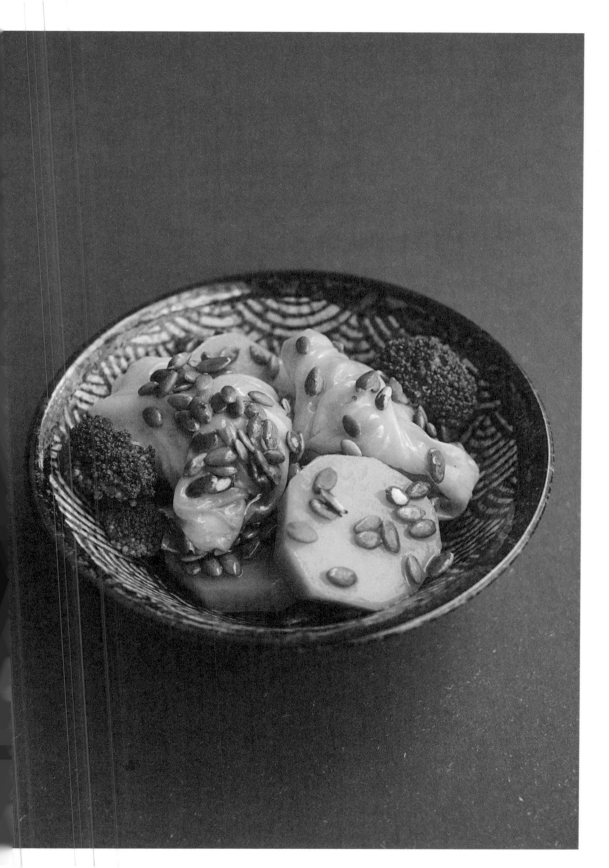

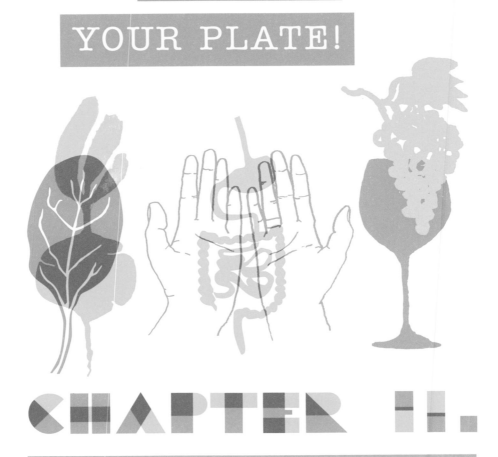

PERK UP YOUR PLATE!

CHAPTER 11.

Learn to find the vintage wine in the vegetable section!

If you eat beetroot your pee takes on a reddish hue. Have you wondered how that's possible?

It would be one thing if your poo was coloured, because that could just be something that had passed through the gut and out again. But for your pee to be red means that the dye must be absorbed by the body and sent around the bloodstream before being cleaned by the kidneys and turned into urine.

Beetroot juice quite simply makes your blood a little bit redder, and marinates your organs. When we eat colourful vegetables, we paint our insides with healthy polyphenols. That's why Niklas and I like colourful food.

The dye pigments are polyphenols, and flavonoids are among the best known sub-groups of these. There are at least 4,000 flavonoids, and new ones are being discovered the whole time. In many studies, flavonoids have been linked to a reduced risk of conditions, including cardiovascular disease.

Researchers were once most interested in the antioxidant effects of polyphenols, but today studies primarily examine how these are used and transformed by the gut bacteria into substances that the body can then absorb and use. This relates to everything from getting the immune system in shape to producing signal substances that help your brain work efficiently.

Are you one of those people who think that tomatoes used to taste better than the watery ones now available in the supermarket?

In 2017 an international research team from the USA, China, Spain and Israel reported that they had investigated 398 traditional tomato varieties and discovered that no fewer than 13 flavour substances had been almost completely eliminated from modern variants.

The once complex wealth of flavours had been replaced by

tomatoes with essentially only two dominant flavour substances.

The flavours had fallen victim to 100 years of cultivation, intended only to achieve larger, longer lasting tomatoes. This is extremely problematic, because research simultaneously shows that the complexity of the flavours reflects the number of beneficial substances and how healthy the tomatoes are to eat.

A few years ago, the Swedish National Food Agency carried out an analysis demonstrating that the degree of ripeness very significantly affected the levels of lycopene in tomatoes – a substance thought to counteract prostate cancer. The riper the tomato, the more lycopene it contains. And not only the cultivation methods, but the practice of picking and selling unripe tomatoes to reduce waste

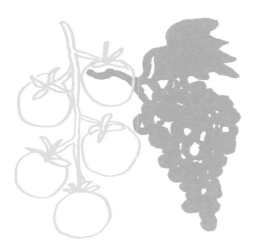

has also contributed to depleting these substances.

There are a number of extensive studies demonstrating that older varieties of both cereals and vegetables contained more varied and richer vitamins and minerals. This also applies to Swedish cereal grains, as made clear in trial cultivations at the Swedish University of Agricultural Sciences, reported as early as 2006. The levels of zinc, a mineral thought to counteract depression, had also fallen.

In this case, the depletion of arable land was indicated as an important cause. But there are other factors that can also play a role.

Have you ever thought about what differentiates a fine wine from a standard one? You might think that the fine wine would have come from the most fertile soil. But on the contrary, it's the mass-produced wines that are cultivated on the best land. In more barren, drier areas, the vines are forced to fight for survival. The grapes are fewer and smaller, but simultaneously absolutely packed with flavonoids and tannins.

The substances that give the wine so much flavour are in fact the plant's own immune defences. These are small chemicals that protect the vine from pests and fungal attacks, and the more the plant is forced to struggle, the better the wine is.

In other words, it's the plant's own protective agents that are then

– usually – so beneficial for us to eat. It's the same with plants that have been cultivated free of toxins, without pesticides. They compensate by producing more of their own protective substances. Plants grown out in the open air also develop more polyphenols (and therefore often have more colour and flavour), to protect themselves against the sun's ultraviolet radiation, than plants grown in a greenhouse.

A group of researchers at the University of Pisa has for several years successfully explored ways of increasing polyphenol content in crops by deliberately stressing them with salt water, strong sunlight and air composition. According to these researchers, the challenge isn't in increasing the polyphenols, but instead in doing so while retaining a high yield from the harvest.

If we once again look at the blue zones where people live to be very old yet still healthy, all of these places are difficult to cultivate and have poor soils. Internationally renowned researcher Craig Wilcox has for many years studied the long-lived people on Okinawa. When I met him during a visit to the Japanese island, he explained that the poor soils meant that the vegetables and herbs making up the inhabitants' diet were extremely nutrient dense.

It's as if all of the vegetables they ever ate had been vintage wines!

The Japanese islanders' gut bacteria have been fed a never-ending supply of microscopic raw materials which they have then been able to convert to hormones and other important signal substances required by humans to be healthy.

In small doses, we become healthier by eating the plants' own defensive substances. But if we were to eat too much, which is almost impossible as long as we eat normal vegetables and avoid the toxic plants that we can't tolerate, we might become sick.

So why are we healthier by eating small doses of something that's actually toxic? Well, it's a bit like a vaccine. In small doses, the toxins stimulate our immune system, but only just enough so that it doesn't nod off.

This effect even has a name. It's called hormesis, and is described quite well in the old saying: "What doesn't kill us makes us stronger."

Some researchers go even further and say that the gut bacteria and cells in our bodies have learned to interpret our existence through the food we eat.

In times when the plants contain more than usual of their own protective products, our second brain in the stomach works out that times are tough and that hunger may be on the way. So that we are prepared for this, our own immune system is activated, entering a reinforced standby mode.

This could explain how it is that our bodies react with the same

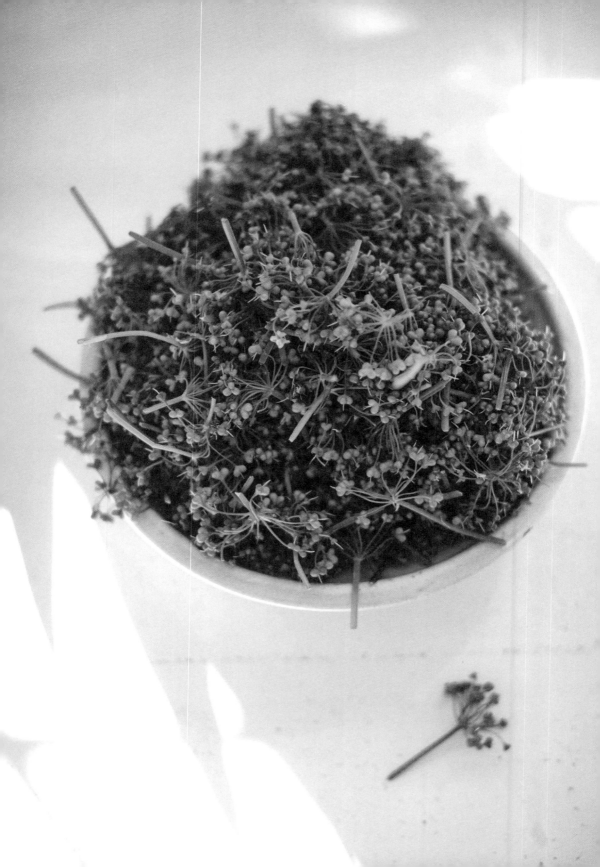

health-promoting defence mechanisms when we are affected by hunger as when we eat particularly nutrient dense food.

Niklas:

That's really interesting, Henrik. Philosophical, even! But now we really should talk about ingredients!

Henrik:

OK, OK. Which is healthiest, a green apple or a red one? Answer: the red one.

The explanation isn't that healthy polyphenols can be found in colourful plants. Instead, the polyphenols are the actual colour.

Try it out yourself next time you go food shopping. Will you choose white or red cabbage? Red or green apples? Yellow or red onions? Ordinary potatoes or blue potatoes? White or black rice? Green or red grapes? Iceberg lettuce or kale? The colours guide you the right way. The stronger the colour, the better.

And a lot of this is on the surface. So eat the skin if you can, and don't remove too many layers of the onion. If you do, you're losing a lot of the healthiest part.

When you look around in nature, of course you see lots of green plants. The reason for the green colour is the chlorophyll, and when this disappears in the autumn, lots of colours are revealed. These were there the whole time, behind the green. Autumn colours are dominated by yellow xanthophyll such as lutein, orange beta-carotene and red anthocyanin.

When we keep recommending leafy green vegetables, it's not just because you need to eat these green colours, but also because such vegetables are extremely rich in the benefits of other colours.

But what about garlic, then? It's white. But surely it's healthy anyway? Yes, and the explanation is that for alliums this light colour is typical. The flavonols quercetin and kaempferol are white or creamy in colour. If you choose red onion, you also get red anthocyanin. But white also belongs on your plate, as does black.

So a good tip is to eat all the colours of the rainbow! And don't forget the greyscale.

On the next page, you can find a simple guide. But there's a lot more to explore, if you're interested. Artists have always strived to refine their knowledge of which plants contain pigments with varying shades. We have many reasons to take inspiration from their work.

Paint your insides – and make yourself happy

Green: leafy green vegetables such as lettuce, spinach and chard. Avocados, courgettes, broccoli, curly kale and herbs like basil.

Green plants are often rich in calcium, folate, vitamin C, flavonoids and antioxidants. Also often contain nitrate.

Red: tomato, red cabbage, red pepper, red onion, lingonberries, beetroot and red apples.

Red plants contain a lot of carotenoids, anthocyanin and also quercetin. Lycopene gives tomatoes their colour. Betalains give the deep red colour to beetroot, but can also provide a yellow pigment.

Yellow: orange, carrot, lemon, squash, turmeric, sweet potato and golden beet.

Yellow plants often contain the carotenoid lutein, which produces a yellow colour, including in egg yolks. Alpha and beta-carotenes give carrots their colour. They are often rich in vitamin C, vitamin E and folate.

Blue/black: blueberries, blackberries, aubergines, olives, black rice and nori seaweed.

Blue plants often contain healthy anthocyanin and other substances.

White: onions, white cabbage, cauliflower, bananas and asparagus.

White plants contain quercetin and kaempferol, together with friendly fibre such as inulin and resistant starch, allicin (onions), calcium, iron, vitamin C and beta-carotene.

It isn't just the colour that indicates the food is healthy. The same applies to smell and flavour.

Think about this for a moment. Why does your breath smell when you've eaten garlic? After all, you swallowed garlic. You didn't breathe it in!

The explanation is that the substances that smell are absorbed in the gut and then travel around in the blood before being secreted in the lungs and travelling out on exhalations.

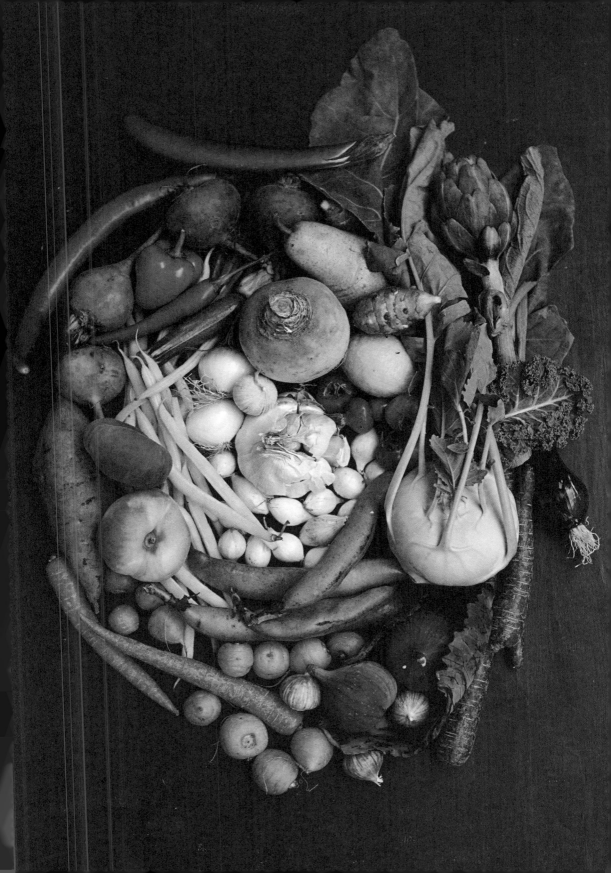

So the garlic smell has impregnated your entire body. Just like plant colourings bathe our internal organs with antioxidants, smells and aromas do the same thing, for the simple reason that it's often the different polyphenols that smell.

Aromatherapy as a treatment for disease has been known since ancient times. Here, essential oils are used, with scents of things like chamomile, rose and lemon. It isn't unreasonable that these could have an effect, not least in terms of stress reduction. Research in this area is very limited, but there are studies showing that the inhalation of several such oils can reduce anxiety.

One fairly well studied example is coffee, where several of the most pleasant aromas have been shown to come from strong antioxidants.

In another study, researchers asked women to smell saffron in a form that was so diluted it wasn't possible to distinguish it consciously. After 20 minutes, these women had fewer stress hormones than the control group and had decreased symptoms of anxiety and worry.

Scents and flavours from food can therefore be described as signals from biologically active substances in the meal. It seems logical that, just like animals, our ancestors could find their way to healthy food using their nose and taste buds.

In fact you can thank the bacteria in the cavity inside your nose for your ability to detect scents. If you have a dry nose, your scent bacteria are depleted and you can detect fewer variations. So you should drink plenty of water before eating a meal so that you can enjoy it properly. Just like strong colours, strong and clear flavours go hand-in-hand with a strong effect on the human body. All herbs are at the top of the list of plants containing the most antioxidants, and these herbs have often been used as natural healing products in teas and compresses.

The healthiest ingredients aren't sweet and ingratiating, but aromatic and have a strong, pungent or bitter and sometimes sour flavour. These are flavours you have to get used to, but which you'll soon find it's difficult to live without.

Boost your body with terrific turmeric

There's a lot of talk about superfoods today – but one thing which is all too rarely discussed is how much our bodies can absorb of the super nutrients that we consume.

Take turmeric, for example. It contains the extremely interesting substance curcumin, which is a polyphenol with a strong anti-inflammatory effect. And if you listen to all the enthusiastic researchers, it can heal almost everything, including stress, anxiety and depression. It even works on many cancers. In animal testing.

Let's repeat that. In animal testing.

In animal testing, curcumin is often injected. Sometimes straight into the brain, mixed with nano particles. In other testing, cancer cells are grown and curcumin is dripped onto them. But when ordinary humans eat turmeric, almost all of the curcumin stops in the gut, and the rest in the liver – and then we pee the rest out. If you take a blood sample afterwards, there's either no curcumin at all or, at best, barely measurable traces.

You might object that in India they've been eating turmeric for thousands of years, and that they know it's good for them.

Yes, but they've been eating curry.

And this brings us to the essential point. It's rarely a good idea to eat superfoods separately. It's much wiser to see how they have been used in traditional cooking, because if we use turmeric the right way, we can get at least some of the positive effects it is alleged to have on health.

And the right way isn't to take a turmeric shot or grate turmeric over a random dish. And definitely not to eat a tablespoon of turmeric powder once a day.

So how do we make it easier for our bodies to access all the good stuff in turmeric? There are three really simple tricks on the following page.

1. Mix it with black pepper. It doesn't seem to be a coincidence that black pepper has long been included in food all around the world. It's also a key component of curry mixes, together with turmeric. Our bodies don't want to consume turmeric, and defend themselves against it – but black pepper contains a substance, piperine, which prevents the breakdown of turmeric that otherwise begins in the gut.

2. Mix it with fat, ideally olive oil. The fat combines with the active substance in the turmeric and protects it from being broken down by enzymes in the gut, and then it can more easily move into the lymphatic system without being captured in the liver.

3. Heat it up. While the turmeric is cold, the body barely absorbs any of it, even if you have done everything right up to this point. The reason is that curcumin isn't at all water-soluble. But we can change this by heating the food. The easiest way is to stir fry or quickly sauté it. Pretty much like they've always done in India. It doesn't need to be any more difficult than that.

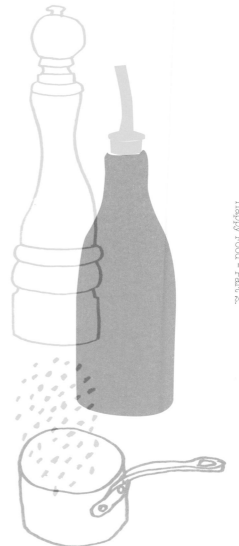

Other top tips

Turmeric isn't the only superfood that must be handled carefully to obtain the promised health benefits. In this book we present a selection of the very best feel-good foods. So we think it's important to give you a few simple rules:

Don't get hung up on ingredients that are called superfoods, even if they may have health benefits. The key to good health is always variation.

Judge superfoods on the basis of the amount you really eat. Don't force yourself to eat something you hate just because it's at the top of the list when you could simply take a bite of another nutritious food you prefer.

Cook your food in different ways. Many vitamins and other healthy substances are destroyed by cooking, while others are released and can more easily be absorbed by the body.

Have both hot and cold dishes on your menu. Cooking your food at really high temperatures may result in the formation of harmful substances that you don't want to expose yourself to every time you eat – perhaps just sometimes for the sake of flavour.

Avoid boiling food in lots of water. Cooking this way means that many (though not all) water-soluble vitamins are lost into the water. Otherwise, it's hard to completely massacre all of the nutrients as long as we're talking about normal cooking in a domestic kitchen.

But processed convenience food is a completely different problem. Here individual ingredients, such as tomatoes, can have been heated during several different production phases, every time losing 10–20% of their healthy load.

Rely on your senses to assess shelf life. There's a lot of exaggeration online. Ignore this and instead rely on your own sight, smell, taste and feeling. Some ingredients such as apples can keep for a long time, while asparagus and broccoli lose a lot of their nutritional value quite quickly. Use your eyes. When broccoli starts to go yellowish grey, you know that the protective vitamin C is on the way out.

The most important thing: Eat! This may seem like ridiculous advice. But it quickly gets confusing if you have to constantly think about the healthiest way to eat a vegetable. The most important thing is simply to eat vegetables as often as you can, and then if you sometimes get a little more or less of any vitamin it really doesn't make much difference overall.

The hottest health trend –
Golden milk

Turmeric has made researchers all around the world turn somersaults from excitement. But to be absorbed by the body, it needs to be cooked in the right way – using heat, fat and protected by black pepper. It's no coincidence that for thousands of years turmeric has been one of the foundations of both Eastern medicine and curry.

serves 4

Golden milk paste:
1 tsp cardamom seeds
1 tsp whole black pepper
2 tbsp ground turmeric
2 tsp ground cinnamon
2 tbsp grated ginger
150 ml water

800 ml milk or plant-based milk
    such as almond or oat milk

1. Grind the cardamom and
    black pepper finely in a mortar
    and pestle.
2. Mix with the other ingredients
    in a saucepan.
3. Bring gently to the boil
    and allow to simmer while
    stirring for 1–2 minutes until
    it has thickened.
4. Heat the milk and add 1–2 tbsp
    golden milk paste or to taste.

TOP TIP! To make ginger juice without a blender, grate the ginger on the fine side of a grater, then squeeze out the juice

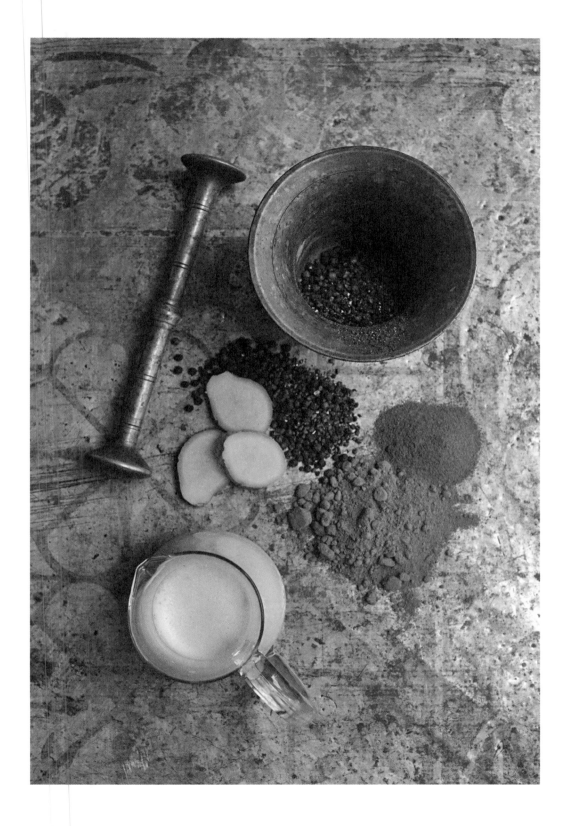

Happy Superfoods

[Colour palette]

Kale: It's not surprising that the kale trend has spread like a forest fire over the last few years. If kale was a multivitamin tablet, it would cover almost every requirement. Among other things, the content of vitamins C and K give an anti-inflammatory boost that is thought to prevent depression. Kale also has properties that can reduce sugar cravings and facilitate weight loss.

But of course the competition is tough in the hyper trendy cruciferous vegetable group, where we also find vitamin C-rich horseradish, folate-packed broccoli and pak choi with its anti-cancer glucosinolates. This family also includes wasabi, cauliflower and white cabbage – in fact most brassicas, including swede and kohlrabi. And don't forget turnip, rocket and radishes, together with rapeseed, mustard and cress. Have I forgotten anything?

Turmeric: One of the most talked-about discoveries in the dietary field in recent years, which in one study was shown to have as strong an effect against depression as the SSRI Fluoxetine (Prozac), although of course this needs to be confirmed by other studies. The active ingredient curcumin is strongly anti-inflammatory and is thought to provide protection against everything from cancer to rheumatoid arthritis. Turmeric is included in traditional curry mixtures and has been part of Eastern medicine for several thousand years. However, it's important to eat turmeric heated and together with both fat and black pepper to improve uptake.

Ginger: Certainly, the health hype is justified. But be cautious. In slightly higher doses, one of the most highly acclaimed superfoods can actually trigger depression!

Ginger has been part of Eastern medicine for at least 4,700 years, and is very important within Indian Ayurvedic medicine. The classic use is to improve digestion and treat wounds, but ginger has a much broader repertoire. Not least its anti-inflammatory effect, which is thought to prevent mental illness.

Studies suggest that the active substances in ginger – mainly gingerols, shogaol and paradol – improve heart health, counteract cancer and metastasis, Type 2 diabetes, stomach and intestinal problems, bronchial infections, asthma and rheumatism. But ginger is a double-edged sword, and if you're over-sensitive there is a risk that it may make you feel worse.

Lingonberries: Nordic super berries, with lingonberries and blueberries at the forefront, are among the most anti-inflammatory foods you can consume. One comparison showed that lingonberries are much healthier than the highly acclaimed acai berry.

According to this study, lingonberries work as a fertiliser for the two superbacteria, Akkermansia and Faecalibacterium. In total, 14 gut bacteria species were affected by lingonberries, and the changes were of the type associated with a reduced risk of developing diabetes.

In animal testing, lingonberries lead to reduced weight, better blood sugar and blood fats, significantly reduced chronic inflammation and sealing of intestinal leakage.

Lingonberries contain high levels of quercetin, which is one of the strongest anti-inflammatory substances found in food, and which protects against depression caused by stress. Blueberries also contain lots of quercetin. The levels are significantly higher in wild blueberries than in cultivated ones, which is what you can most often buy.

Quercetin is also present in other dark berries such as blackcurrants, blackberries and sea buckthorn. But the very highest concentrations are actually found in capers and lovage. They contain ten times as much quercetin as wild blueberries, but of course it's more difficult to eat as much of them.

Black pepper: The active substance is called piperine, and it has been shown by studies to have as strong an antidepressant effect as several common medicines, even at doses of around half a gram per day! The uptake of the active substance in turmeric increases by 2,000% if taken with black pepper. Chilli pepper and cayenne pepper are also believed to be able to reduce anxiety and worry, but the effect is nothing like as strong as for normal black pepper.

Cinnamon: Bursting with antioxidants, cinnamon has a strong anti-inflammatory effect. But it's cinnamon's ability to influence insulin sensitivity and thus counteract both weight gain and Type 2 diabetes that makes it most interesting. It's probably also this effect that means cinnamon has also been shown to protect the brain and our mental abilities. The active substance coumarin is present in all cinnamon, but most of all in cassia or Chinese cinnamon. However, coumarin can cause liver damage in excess, so a maximum of 1.5 teaspoons per day for an adult is advised.

Kale salad with Parmesan and basil gremolata

Kale has an undeserved bad reputation because of its slightly stringy consistency. In the recipe below, we use a simple chef's trick to get the leaves to soften.

serves 4

200 g kale, shredded
2 tsp salt
1 bunch basil
1 lemon
3 tbsp olive oil
4 tbsp grated Parmesan cheese

1. Mix the shredded kale and 1½ tsp salt. Knead gently until the kale becomes darker in colour and releases a little liquid.
2. Grind the basil, the peel of 1 lemon, ½ tsp salt and 1 tbsp olive oil using a mortar and pestle.
3. Mix the kale, grated Parmesan and remaining olive oil, and top with the basil dressing.

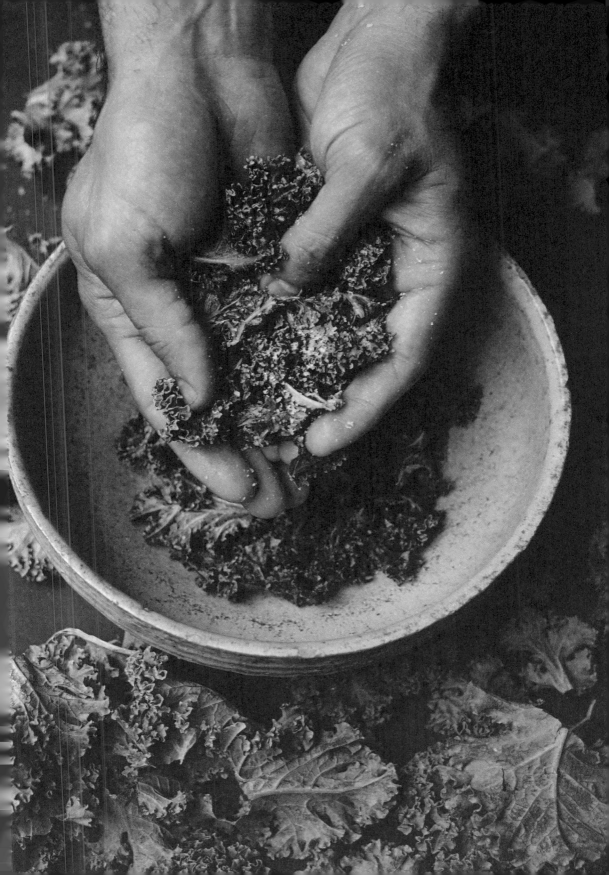

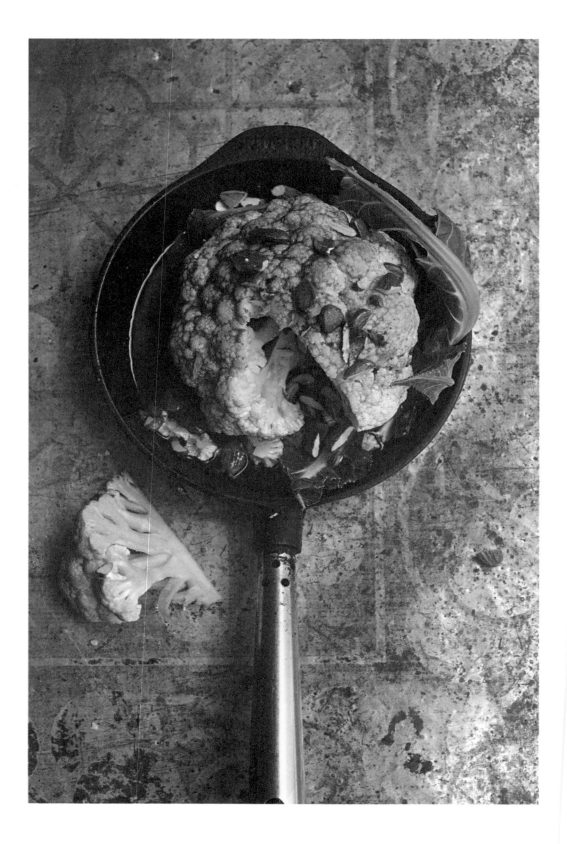

Curry roasted whole cauliflower and almonds

Cauliflower is often, and undeservedly, sidelined by other hyped foods such as kale and broccoli. Perhaps this is because of its white colour. But cauliflower is an undervalued source of vitamins, minerals, polyphenols and fibre which nourishes the gut flora. Try eating both raw and lightly cooked (ideally steamed rather than boiled in lots of water). Once cooked, cauliflower binds gall, which is linked to positive effects on the heart. Raw cauliflower preserves more of the healthy glucosinolates. So vary how you prepare it!

serves 4

1–2 cauliflowers
3 tbsp coconut oil
2 tbsp curry powder
1 tsp salt
2 tbsp almonds, coarsely chopped

1. Preheat oven to 175°C.
2. Wash the cauliflower in cold water and pat dry.
3. Mix the coconut oil, curry powder and salt.
4. Rub the spice mix into the cauliflower, making sure you use it all.
5. Place in an ovenproof dish and bake in the oven until the cauliflower is soft in the centre. Use a skewer or narrow-bladed knife to test. If it gets too brown before it's cooked through, cover it with aluminium foil and reduce the oven temperature to 150°C.
6. Toast the almonds in a pan and serve sprinkled over the cauliflower.

Fried pickled herring with potato salad, lingonberries and parsley

Pickled herring is a classic Nordic dish. One small piece of herring contains as much healthy omega-3 as an expensive capsule from a health food shop. Your brain largely consists of this type of fat. Here your gut bacteria can also indulge in resistant starch, and lots of the healthy substances found in lingonberries and parsley. And it also tastes great! Please sir, I want some more.

serves 4

4–8 salted herring
2–3 eggs
100 g buckwheat flour
200 g almond flour
3–4 tbsp butter
3 tbsp lingonberries, fresh or
     frozen
2 tbsp chopped parsley
1 tbsp coarse grain mustard
Potato salad, see recipe on
     page 109

1. Soak the fish according to the manufacturer's instructions.
2. Dry on paper.
3. Break the eggs into a bowl and whisk.
4. Roll the fish in the buckwheat flour, then in the egg, and finally in the almond flour.
5. Fry in butter over a medium heat until golden brown, about 2-4 minutes on each side.
6. Remove the fish from the pan and place on a serving dish.
7. Remove the pan from the heat and add the lingonberries, parsley and mustard.
8. Stir and add the lingonberry mixture on top of the fish. Serve with potato salad and a little brown butter to taste, if liked.

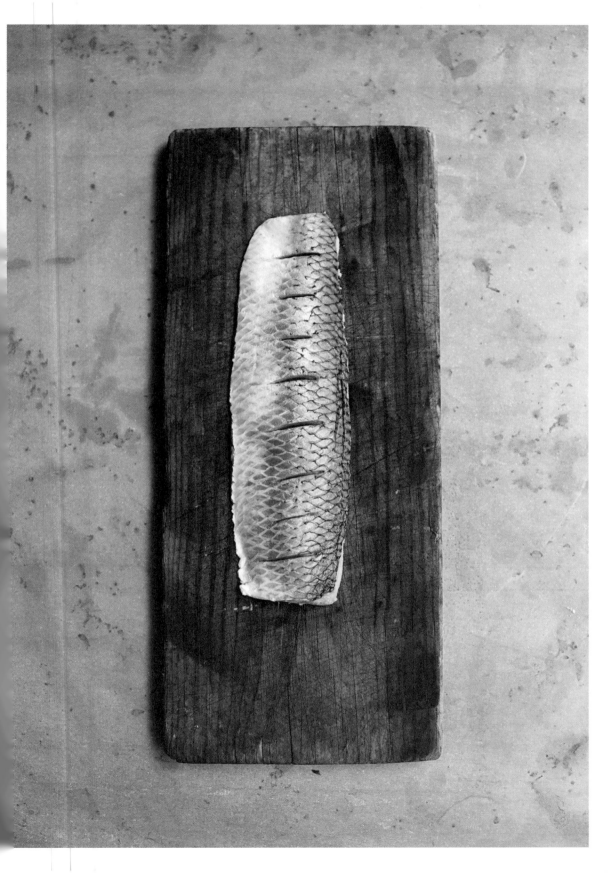

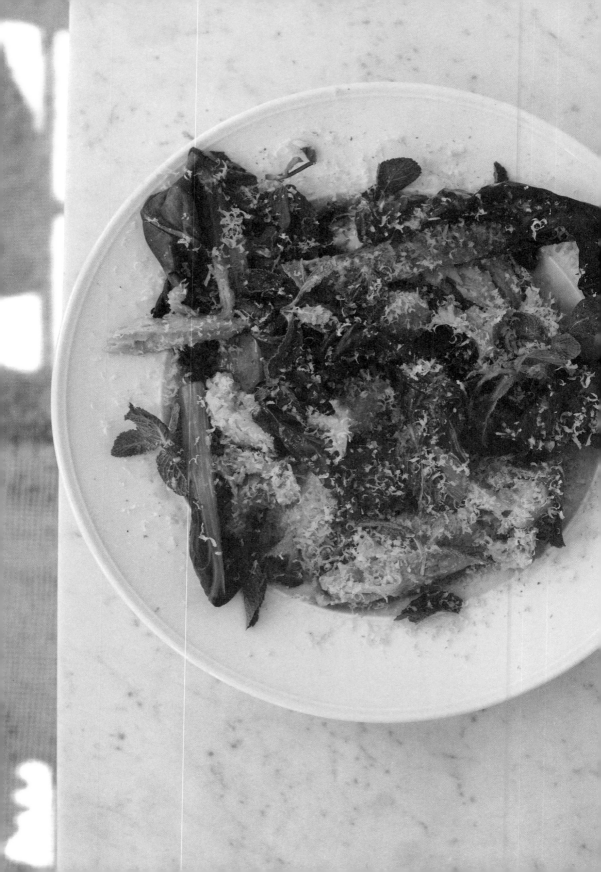

Sweet potato with chard, garlic, olive oil and walnuts

This dish doesn't merely taste great. It's a survival kit for a future traveller to the planet Mars. Chard is one of the plants that was evaluated early on as ideal for taking on long journeys in space. And sweet potato is a nutrient booster that's routinely used as a famine relief crop. Add to this garlic, a good quality olive oil and walnuts, and it makes you happy just to read about it!

serves 4

3–4 sweet potatoes
3 tbsp olive oil
100 g walnuts
1 bunch chard leaves
2 garlic cloves, peeled

1. Preheat the oven to 175°C.
2. Cut the sweet potatoes in half.
3. Grease an ovenproof dish with a little olive oil and place the sweet potatoes in it, cut side down.
4. Bake in the oven for about 45 minutes.
5. Toast the walnuts in a pan over a medium heat.
6. Steam the chard leaves for 1–2 minutes until soft or boil quickly in lightly salted water.
7. Chop the garlic and sauté in olive oil quickly over a medium heat.
8. Toss the chard with the garlic and serve with sweet potatoes and toasted walnuts.

Our banana ice cream

A modern classic. Unripened green bananas are packed with resistant starch. And they're also convenient to store in the freezer!

serves 4

4 bananas

1. Peel and slice the bananas, then freeze.
2. Blend the frozen bananas in a food processor to a creamy consistency.
3. Now they're ready to eat!

- - - - - - - - - - - - - - - - - - - -

TOP TIP! Experiment with flavours such as fresh mango or cocoa. Find your own favourite topping; toasted coconut flakes, cocoa nibs, roasted hazelnuts, honey etc.

- - - - - - - - - - - - - - - - - - - -

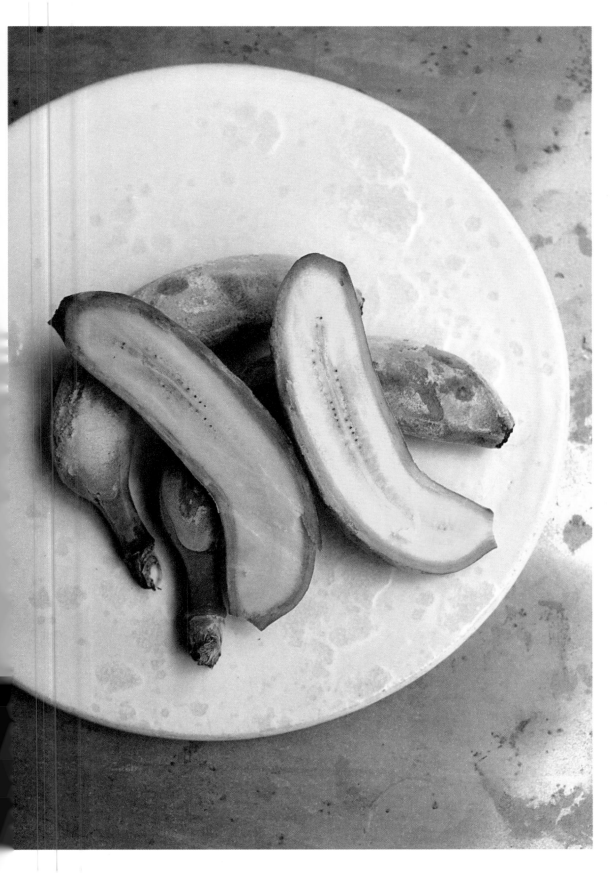

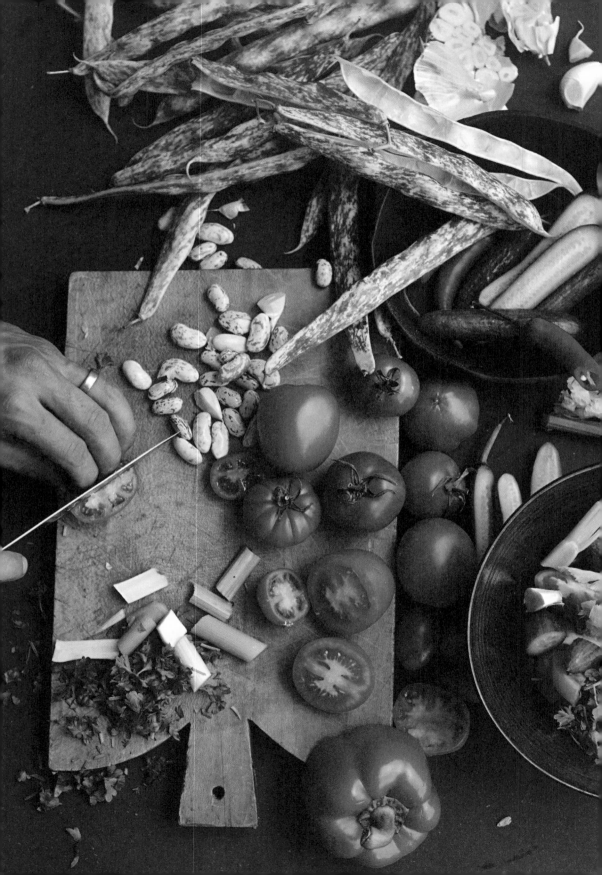

Gazpacho

A fresh gazpacho with a little zing always stimulates the mind! Strong spices such as chilli are good for your health, but we'd like to give an extra big cheer for standard freshly ground black pepper. It contains piperine, a substance that in experiments has had an equally good effect as antidepressant medications, even at doses of only half a gram of freshly ground black pepper a day.

serves 4

1 red pepper
1 red chilli
1–2 cloves of garlic
1 shallot
½ cucumber
3–4 large tomatoes
1 bunch basil
200 ml vegetable stock
1 tbsp lemon juice
tabasco, to taste
3 tbsp olive oil
seea salt and freshly ground black
        pepper

1. Deseed the pepper and chilli.
2. Peel the garlic, shallot and cucumber.
3. Coarsely chop all the vegetables and mix in a blender with the other ingredients until smooth.
4. Leave in the refrigerator for 1 hour.
5. If necessary, season with more salt, black pepper, lemon juice and tabasco.

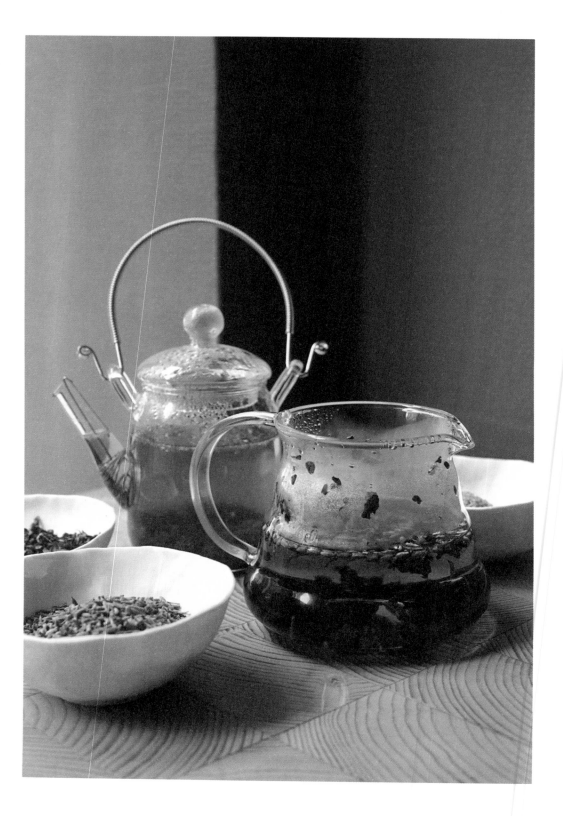

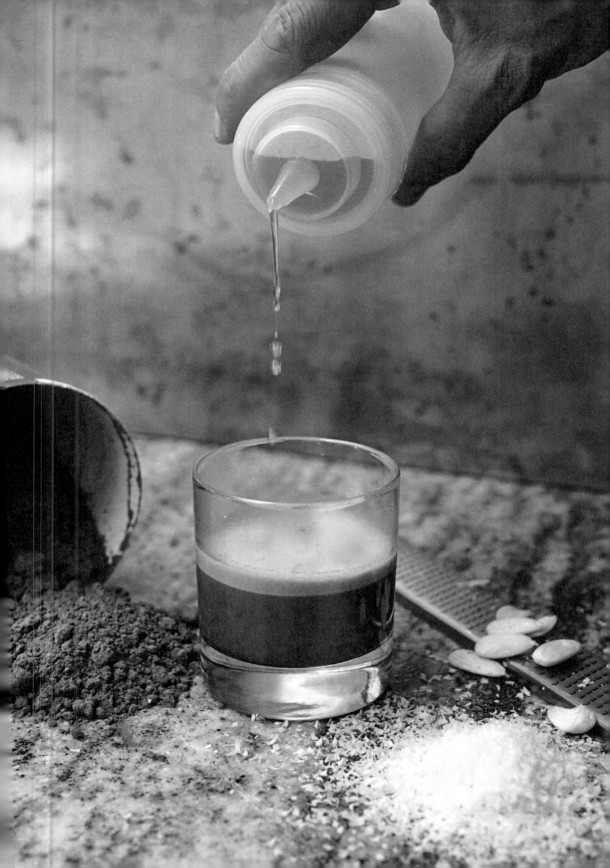

Hot chocolate

Cocoa increases the hormones that regulate happiness and satisfaction, and also love. This is perfect to snuggle up with on the sofa when it's grey and miserable out.

serves 4

800 ml milk or plant-based milk
    such as almond or oat milk
2 tbsp cocoa
½ tsp ground cardamom
1 tbsp honey or agave syrup

1. Heat the milk.
2. Add the other ingredients and whisk to a smooth mixture.
3. Leave to stand for 4–6 minutes.
4. Add more honey if required.

Salt-roasted pumpkin seeds

Make your own happy snacks! Pumpkin seeds aren't only full of tryptophan, a precursor to the happiness hormone serotonin. They also contain lots of zinc and magnesium, shortages of which can contribute to depression.

serves 4

200 g pumpkin seeds
1 tbsp salt
2 tbsp water

1. Toast the pumpkin seeds in a frying pan over a medium heat.
2. When they have browned and darkened slightly and started to sweat a little, add the salt and water.
3. Stir and allow to boil dry.
4. Pour onto a plate and serve as a snack.

- - - - - - - - - - - - - - - - - - -

TOP TIP! These can be flavoured, for example with ground fennel seed or caraway. In this case, add about 1 teaspoon at the same time as the salt. Great for topping a stew or salad.

- - - - - - - - - - - - - - - - - - -

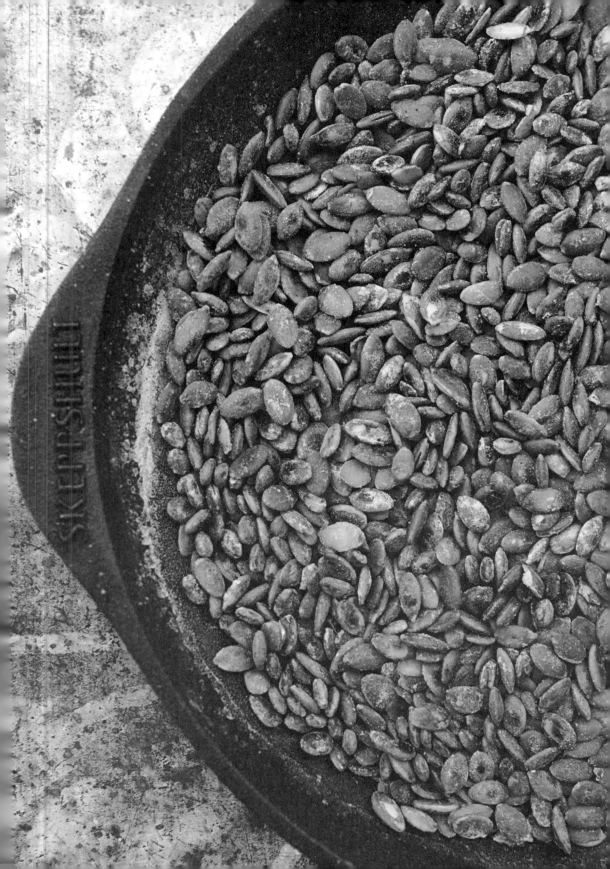

Linseed crackers with Roquefort, walnuts and honey

Unpasteurised cheese is one of the few ways to easily consume living bacterial cultures. They provide virtually the same set of lactobacilli as an expensive capsules, but they taste so much better! If you know a beekeeper, make sure you get hold of fresh honey, which is chock-full of lactic acid bacteria, during the first two weeks. Nature at its very best!

serves 4

250 g linseeds
50 g sesame seeds
100 g pumpkin seeds
100 g sunflower seeds
350 ml water
1 tbsp sea salt
1 handful walnuts
3 tbsp honey
200 g Roquefort or other
    unpasteurised blue cheese

1. Mix the seeds together, pour on the water and leave in a cool place for 4 hours. Stir once an hour.
2. Preheat the oven to 125°C.
3. Spread the seed pulp in a thin, even layer on a baking sheet covered with baking paper.
4. Sprinkle over the salt.
5. Bake in the middle of the oven for 1 hour. Leave the oven door open a couple of centimetres, or open it every 10 minutes to let out the steam.
6. Reduce the temperature and bake for a further hour.
7. Allow to cool and break into pieces.
8. Serve with walnuts, honey and blue cheese.

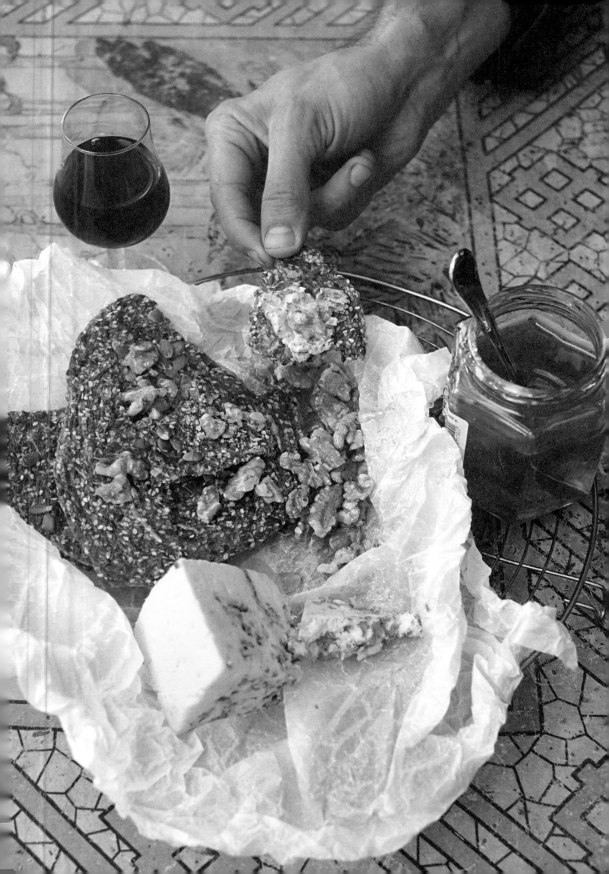

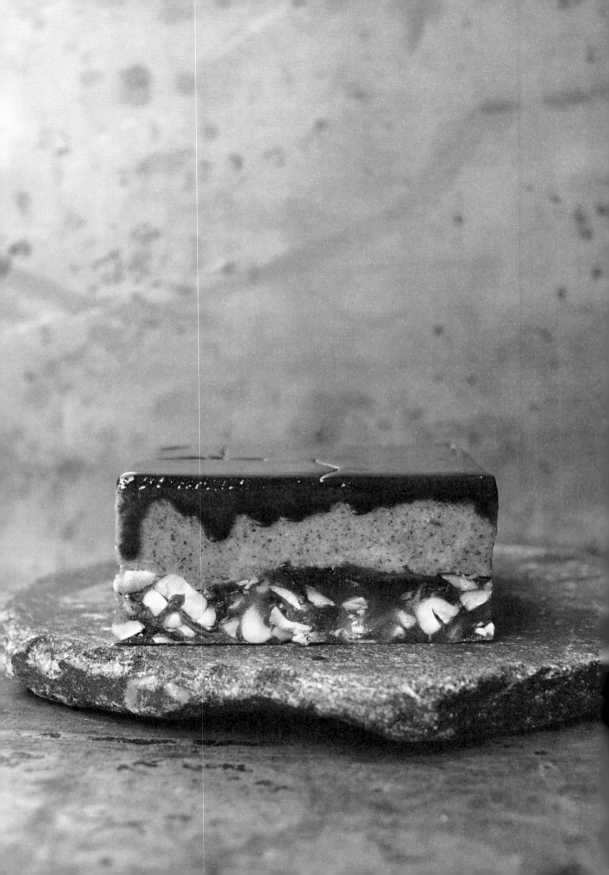

Raw food bar with cocoa, nuts and dates

Why not combine an energy boost with friendly fibre? Medjool dates (the slightly larger variety) are considered not only to be one of the sweeteners that we can best cope with, but are also packed with resistant starch, which provides food for the hungry bacteria that help you to balance your blood sugar.

serves 8–12

Base:
100 g almonds, peeled
100 g cashew nuts
200 g medjool dates, stoned

Filling:
100 ml cashew butter, see recipe
    on page 92
100 ml cold-pressed coconut oil
200 g medjool dates, stoned

Topping:
4 tbsp cold-pressed coconut oil
2 tbsp cocoa

Base:
1. Coarsely chop the nuts.
2. Blend with the dates.
3. Lay in a baking tin coated with cling film. The base should be around 1.5 cm high.
4. Leave in the fridge for 1 hour.

Filling:
5. Blend the cashew butter, coconut oil and dates to a smooth batter.
6. Remove the baking tin from the refrigerator and spread the filling on top of the base.

7. Place in the freezer and allow to stand for at least 1 hour.

Topping:
8. Melt the coconut oil and whisk the cocoa into it.
9. Pour over the filling, covering the whole surface.
10. Leave in the freezer for 1 hour.
11. Remove from the freezer and cut into portions.
12. Allow to stand for a few minutes at room temperature before serving.

Boiled langoustines with saffron mayonnaise

Cheer yourself up with a seafood treat! This dish contains a lot of tryptophan – the precursor to the happiness hormone serotonin – and also important minerals. Saffron can be expensive, but tests have shown that the smell alone can relieve anxiety and depression.

serves 4

12–20 langoustines
2 tbsp salt per litre of water
2 tsp sugar per litre of water
1 bunch crown dill

Saffron Mayonnaise:
0.5 g saffron
1 tbsp Cognac
1 garlic clove, peeled
2 egg yolks
2 tsp French mustard
2 tsp lemon juice
200 ml neutral olive oil

1. Fill a pan with enough water to cover the langoustines and bring to the boil, along with the salt, sugar and crown dill.
2. Place the langoustines in the boiling water and cook for 3–5 minutes depending on size.
3. Remove the langoustines when the cooking time is over. Save and cool the cooking liquid.
4. When the liquid has cooled, add the langoustines back into the liquid and store in the refrigerator for 1–4 days before serving.

Saffron Mayonnaise:
5. Mix the saffron and Cognac and allow to stand for a few minutes.
6. Grate the garlic.
7. Mix the saffron and garlic with the egg yolks, mustard and lemon juice.
8. Add the oil a little at a time, continuing to whisk.
9. Serve the saffron mayonnaise with the boiled langoustines.

- - - - - - - - - - - - - - - - - - - -

TOP TIP! Mix the langoustines with lobster, crab, crayfish and prawns.

- - - - - - - - - - - - - - - - - - - -

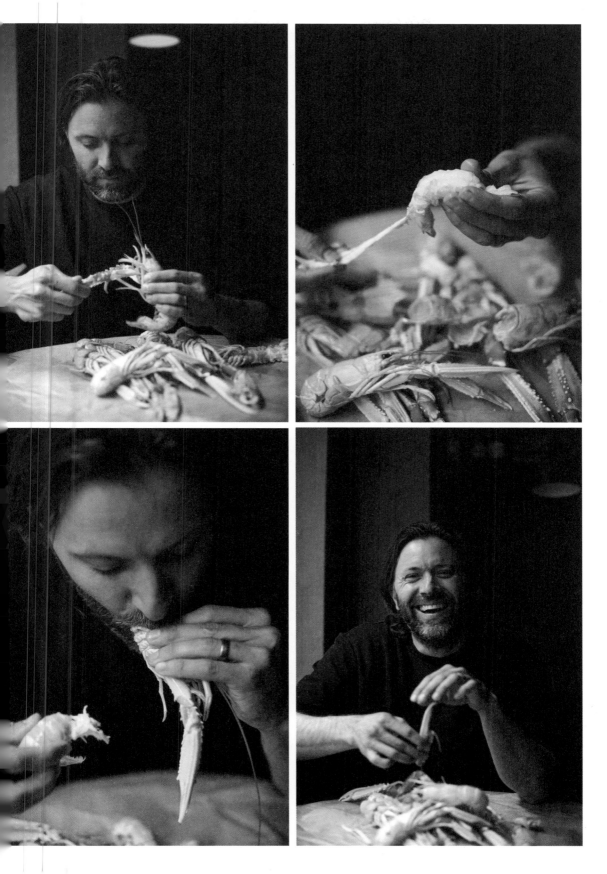

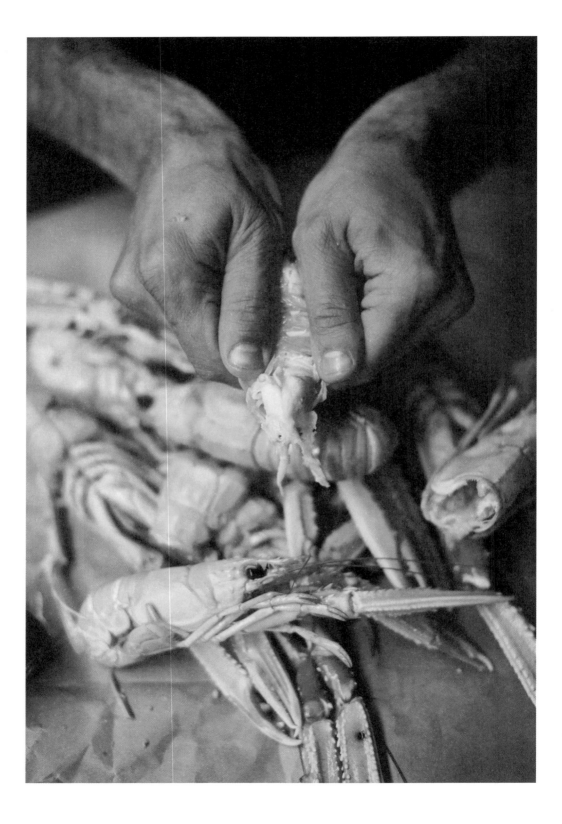

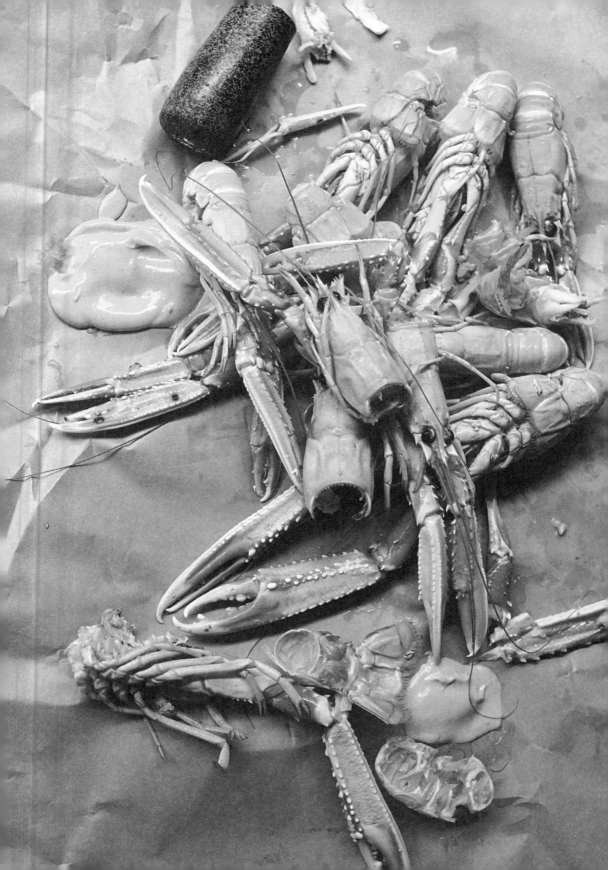

Happy Superfoods

[Happiness pills]

Pumpkin seeds: A genuine happy seed! Pumpkin seeds are full of tryptophan, a precursor to the happiness hormone serotonin. Pumpkin seeds are also the best source of magnesium (after mineral salts, which we can't really eat much of). Almost one in three Swedes lacks magnesium, which has a clear link to depression.

Pumpkin seeds' three-stage strike against sadness is completed by the fact that the seeds are one of the best sources of zinc, the other mineral deficiency linked to depression.

Vary with other seeds. Pretty much all of them are rich in minerals, vitamins and fibre. You can find lots of tryptophan in squash seeds. Second most can be found in chia, sesame and sunflower seeds. Other sources are beans, lentils, oats and things like spinach and broccoli, together with meat, fish and shellfish.

Dark chocolate: Select chocolate with a cocoa content of at least 70%, not a sweet version. Cocoa contains a large number of flavonoids and other substances that are linked to better brain function and a feeling of well-being. The exact mechanisms aren't yet understood, but cocoa can help to increase both serotonin and dopamine, the signal substance and hormone that regulate happiness and satisfaction. Dark chocolate also contains phenylethylamine, the same substance that's formed when we fall in love. It also counteracts the effects of the stress hormone cortisol. We aren't recommending a purely chocolate diet, but the benefits of a maximum of 40 grams per day seem to outweigh the disadvantages.

Herbal tea: Many different teas can have a positive effect on the health. St John's Wort affects the hormones serotonin, dopamine and noradrenaline and in studies has produced as good an effect as standard antidepressant medications. In other studies, chamomile tea has also been successful as an alternative to standard medication for both anxiety and depression.

An extensive review recently showed that tea drinkers have almost 40% lower risk of depression.

Oysters: One of life's great joys, according to many people. Including health researchers. Here we have nature's own alternative to an antidepressant multivitamin tablet. Approximately seven oysters contain 720% of the recommended daily dose of vitamin B12, 500% of the dose of zinc and 120% of the daily selenium we require, together with half of our daily iron requirement and a good helping of vitamin D, together with various other B vitamins. Contributes both to reducing inflammation in the brain and to balancing the mood hormones serotonin and dopamine. But make sure they were fished from clean water!

Spinach: Never a health top ten without spinach. This green crop is also rich in tryptophan. Chinese leaf and kale are also high up on the list. As is broccoli. Broccoli is a constant!

Beans and lentils: Also packed with tryptophan, but contain more protein. In tofu made from soya beans, the concentration is particularly high, as well as in soy sauce, especially tamari sauce.

Oats: Have a high tryptophan content, as well as wheat bran and wheat germ.

Cheese: We're talking about mature, tasty cheeses such as Parmesan, mozzarella, Gruyère, Edam and Cheddar. Yum. Even just thinking about them makes you happy!

Game: In terms of meat, game is in a class of its own when it comes to high levels of tryptophan. On the throne, we find the king of the forest – the elk. Goat meat comes in a good second place.

Fish and shellfish: High levels of tryptophan in prawns, crabs, lobster and fish like halibut. Salmon also has reasonably high levels. Most seafood helps to perk up the senses.

Egg: Lots of tryptophan, but also angry competitors who counteract uptake. The tryptophan is mainly found in the egg white.

Mushrooms: Exotic mushrooms like shiitake have become trendy in recent years, but normal large mushrooms (portobello) are absolutely fine.

Mustard: If the flavour alone doesn't wake you up, the rush of tryptophan soon will do.

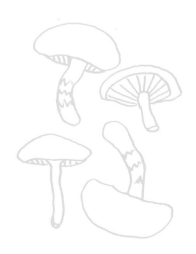

MAKE YOUR GUT HAPPY WITH THE NEW NITRATE TREND

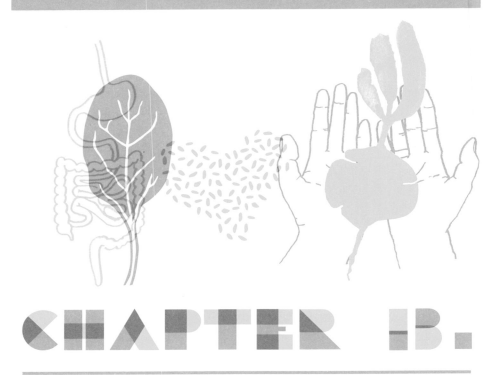

CHAPTER B.

Rejuvenate your brain vessels with nitrate

What we eat affects our health and how we feel, and can have an effect incredibly quickly! It's not a long drawn-out process. If we could look into our cells with an electron microscope, we would see that they are constantly alternating between ageing and rejuvenating depending on the challenges we expose them to.

The eye opener for me was retired doctor and researcher Olle Haglund's beetroot juice.

It transformed me into a 56-year-old in a 21-year-old body, in just a few days.

At least, according to the biological age of my arteries.

I happily go along with British scientist Thomas Sydenham, who in the 1600s coined the expression: "A man is as old as his arteries." Thomas Sydenham wasn't just anyone. He is often called the father of British medicine.

It was also Olle Haglund who introduced me to the technique used to determine the age of arteries. For several years, he has used a measuring device known as an arteriograph, which measures arterial stiffness. Researchers often use these, but normal health centres can rarely afford them.

As we age, our blood vessels become stiff. If this takes place from inside, it is called atherosclerosis. If it takes place in the muscle layer around the vessels, it is called arterial stiffness. This is an invisible disorder that can contribute to stroke and heart attack, without warning. The condition is driven by inflammation in the fatty tissue surrounding the vessel. In other words, just the type of chronic inflammation that starts in the gut.

Half of all Swedes die of cardiovascular diseases, and arterial stiffness is a precursor to high blood pressure, but also to stroke and dementia.

Arterial stiffness can be measured by sending pulse waves into the aorta. And it can also be treated by revising our diet.

For several years, Olle Haglund has experimented with beetroot juice on his patients, and has achieved rather startling results.

A retired professor who had drunk beetroot juice told me that he had reduced his arterial age by 42 years. But at the same time he had stopped consuming sugar and white bread.

Personally, after a few days of juice drinking, my aorta had rejuvenated by a magical 35 years. I also reduced sugar and white bread and ate Mediterranean-inspired food.

A middle-aged woman who, despite regular exercise and normal weight, initially had a 85-year-old's blood vessels, succeeded in reducing her value to that of a 30-year-old, just by changing her diet.

I was later in contact with several other patients who had also succeeded in dramatically reducing their arterial age. A fit 63-year-old eventually achieved the reference value for a 25-year-old.

The underlying theory is an old one. Nitroglycerin has been used against angina since 1867, and in 1998 the Nobel Prize was awarded to researchers who were able to demonstrate that the effect is a result of the fact that nitric oxide gas forms in the vessel wall, where it softens the vessel.

Since then, researchers at a number of institutes have discovered that nitrate-rich vegetables reduce the blood pressure in a manner comparable to medicines, and that the bacterial flora in both the mouth and gut play an important role in the positive effect. So watch out for antibacterial mouthwash too!

By eating nitrate-rich leafy green vegetables such as rocket, spinach, chard and nettles – in other words exactly like our ancestors did – we can stimulate blood vessel function. The fact is that leafy green vegetables constantly stand out as beneficial in all possible dietary research studies.

But the nitrate source that has been most and best explored is still beetroot. It also contains high levels of antioxidants – called betalains – which are required to form nitric oxide.

This is why beetroot juice is frequently used by cyclists and skiers who want to improve their performance. When the nitrate in the beetroot is transformed into nitric oxide, the blood vessels become softer and expand, so the body needs less oxygen to function.

A natural form of doping, you could say.

Because nitrogen expands the very narrowest vessels, the Nobel prize-winning discovery rapidly resulted in a number of potency enhancers. Sigh… Doping and sex are clearly what drives pharmaceutical development, not trying to save lives.

But nitrate can perk you up in more ways than one. In 2015 researchers reported that nitrate-rich vegetables protect the intestinal mucosa and prevent inflammation in the gut. Nitrate quite simply works as an effective fertiliser for a healthy gut flora, so perhaps this is one of the secrets behind the fact that leafy green vegetables are so good for us.

In 2017 it was also reported that beetroot juice contributes to improved brain function by facilitating blood flow and oxygenation in the finely branched vessels of the brain. Above all, nitrate seems to be able to help improve decision-making function, such as not becoming stressed when faced with a choice. This is often associated with hyperactivity and ADHD.

Our top tip is to mix lingonberries with the beetroot juice. This facilitates the conversion of nitrate into nitrogen. The juice also tastes better. And, at the risk of nagging: don't forget leafy green vegetables! They are also bursting with nitrate.

6 benefits of nitrate

1. Reduces blood pressure: A glass of beetroot juice a day gives the same effect as several blood pressure reduction medicines.

2. The gut: Protects the intestinal mucosa and thereby counteracts inflammation in the gut.

3. The brain: Increases blood flow and is thought to be able to counteract dementia. Improve decision-making function in all age groups, which is thought to reduce anxiety.

4. Sex drive: Increases blood flow in the genital organs and thereby increases sex drive. The science underlying this is the basis for several potency enhancers.

5. The heart: Reduces the risk of cardiovascular disease and stroke.

6. Better endurance: Increases oxygen absorption capacity so the muscles operate more efficiently.

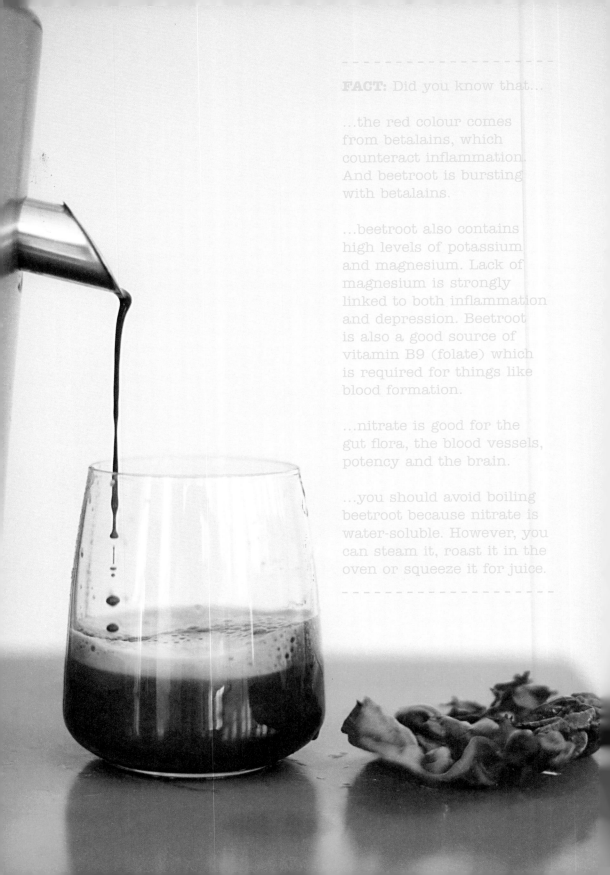

FACT: Did you know that...

...the red colour comes from betalains, which counteract inflammation. And beetroot is bursting with betalains.

...beetroot also contains high levels of potassium and magnesium. Lack of magnesium is strongly linked to both inflammation and depression. Beetroot is also a good source of vitamin B9 (folate) which is required for things like blood formation.

...nitrate is good for the gut flora, the blood vessels, potency and the brain.

...you should avoid boiling beetroot because nitrate is water-soluble. However, you can steam it, roast it in the oven or squeeze it for juice.

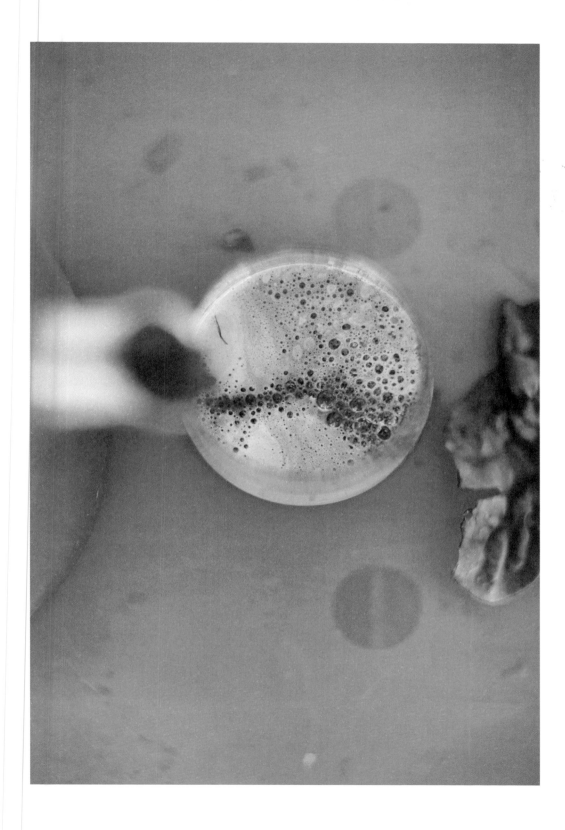

Beetroot, spinach and ginger juice

Leafy green vegetables are another good source of nitrate.

To achieve the best effects in the body, nitrate should be combined with antioxidants, and there are a lot of these in beetroot, spinach and ginger.

serves 4

4–6 large beetroot
1 bunch spinach
4 cm fresh ginger

1. Peel and cut the beetroot and ginger into smaller pieces.
2. Rinse the spinach in cold water.
3. Centrifuge or blend all ingredients into juice.

Olle Haglund's lingonberry and beetroot juice

A real rejuvenation remedy – literally. Henrik's arteries became as elastic as those of a 21-year-old after just a couple of weeks of drinking 100 ml of freshly squeezed beetroot juice every morning.

The Nobel prize-winning discovery that nitrate in foods such as beetroot can expand the blood vessels may be an effective remedy for both high blood pressure and premature ageing.

serves 4

200 ml beetroot juice
200 g lingonberries, fresh or frozen

1. Blend.
2. Drink!

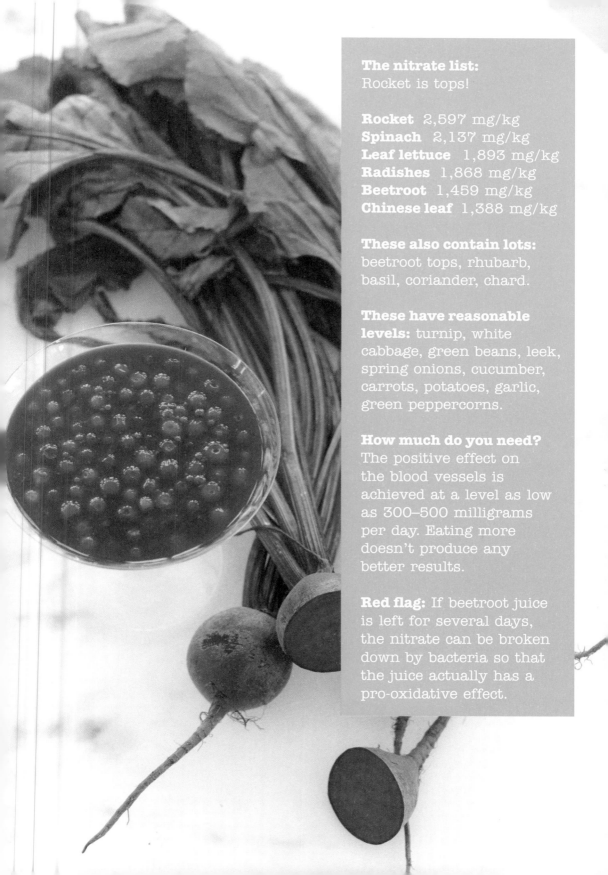

The nitrate list:
Rocket is tops!

Rocket 2,597 mg/kg
Spinach 2,137 mg/kg
Leaf lettuce 1,893 mg/kg
Radishes 1,868 mg/kg
Beetroot 1,459 mg/kg
Chinese leaf 1,388 mg/kg

These also contain lots:
beetroot tops, rhubarb,
basil, coriander, chard.

**These have reasonable
levels:** turnip, white
cabbage, green beans, leek,
spring onions, cucumber,
carrots, potatoes, garlic,
green peppercorns.

How much do you need?
The positive effect on
the blood vessels is
achieved at a level as low
as 300–500 milligrams
per day. Eating more
doesn't produce any
better results.

Red flag: If beetroot juice
is left for several days,
the nitrate can be broken
down by bacteria so that
the juice actually has a
pro-oxidative effect.

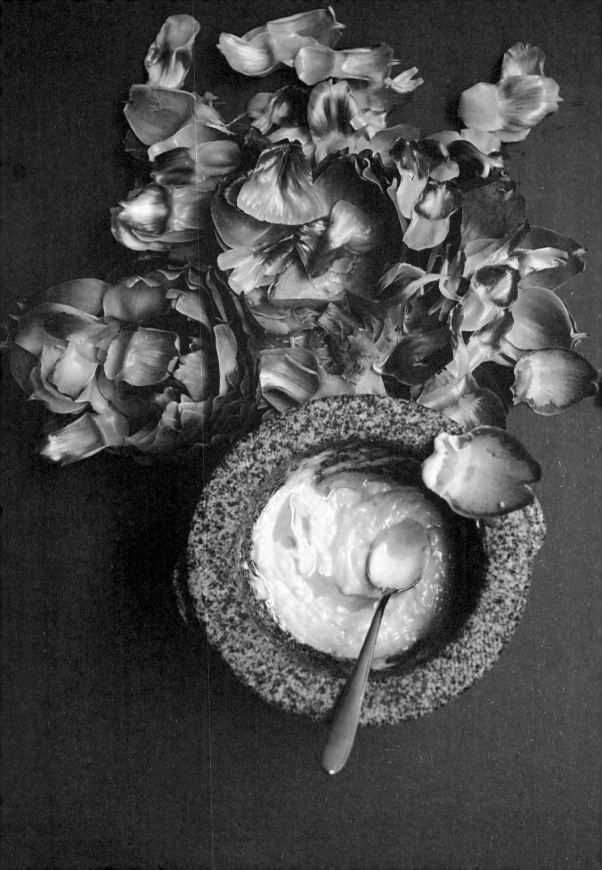

Globe artichokes with aioli

A quick online search will reveal lots of information about Jerusalem artichokes being a good source of healthy inulin fibre. Significantly fewer sources point out that the same fibre is found in abundance in globe artichokes. It's the inulin that gives them the sweet taste. Inulin fibres above all fertilise friendly bifidobacteria, thereby contributing to the production of healing butyric acid.

serves 4

2–4 globe artichokes
1 lemon
2 tbsp salt

Aioli:
1 floury potato
1 garlic clove, peeled
1 egg yolk
2 tsp French mustard
2 tsp lemon juice
150 ml neutral olive oil

1. Cut the stem off the globe artichokes.
2. Cut the lemon in half and place in a saucepan with the globe artichokes and salt.
3. Top up with water. Place a plate, with a diameter slightly smaller than that of the saucepan, on the globe artichokes. It should hold them under the water.
4. Bring to the boil and simmer gently for about 40 minutes or until the lower large leaves are easy to remove.
5. Turn off the heat.
6. Serve them freshly cooked or save and allow to cool in the liquid, before reheating to serve.

Aioli:
7. Peel the potato and boil it until soft in lightly salted water. Allow to cool.
8. Grate the garlic and the cold boiled potato.
9. Mix with the egg yolk, mustard and lemon juice.
10. Add the oil one drop at a time, continuing to whisk.
11. Season with salt and more grated garlic if required.
12. Serve the aioli with warm globe artichoke – remove a leaf and dip it in the aioli.

Make your gut happy with the new nitrate trend

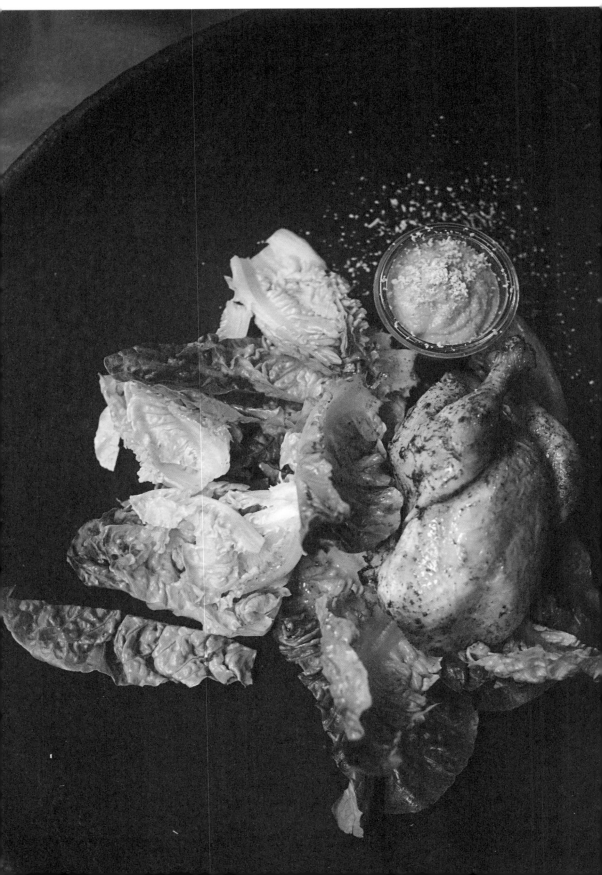

Roast chicken with mojo rojo, almonds and fried lettuce

Fennel and bay leaves are among our forgotten health heroes. The peppery mojo rojo sauce goes well with most things. If you use chicken for this recipe, make it organic because the meat contains healthy fatty acids.

serves 4

1 large chicken or 4 poussins
    of 350 g
200 ml water
1 tbsp chicken stock
1 red chilli
2 shallots, peeled
2 garlic cloves, peeled
½ bulb of fennel
100 ml olive oil
2 bay leaves
2 tsp fennel seeds
2 grilled red peppers
2 tbsp sherry vinegar
5 tbsp almond flour
4 little gem lettuces
3 tbsp coarsely chopped almonds
sea salt

1. Preheat oven to 225°C.
2. Rub the chicken with salt.
3. Place the chicken in an ovenproof dish and put in the oven for 20 minutes.
4. Reduce the heat to 175°C, pour the water and chicken stock over the chicken and continue to cook until the interior temperature is 70°C. Takes about 30 minutes.
5. Baste the chicken every 5 minutes.
6. Remove the chicken from the oven and allow to rest for 10 minutes before carving it.
7. Deseed the chilli.
8. Chop the chilli, shallots, garlic and fennel. Place in a saucepan with olive oil, bay leaves and fennel seeds.
9. Cook until soft over a medium-high heat. Remove from the heat and allow to cool.
10. Add the pepper and sherry vinegar and mix until smooth in a blender or with a stick blender.
11. Add the almond flour and allow to swell for 30 minutes.
12. Cut the lettuces in two and rinse then allow to drip dry.
13. Fry cut side down over a high heat.
14. Serve the fried lettuce with roast chicken and paprika sauce.

Steak tartare with pine nuts, Parmesan, rocket and olive oil

Most people eat too much meat, both in terms of what the body needs and what the planet can cope with. So reduce your portion size and combine it with other things on your plate. The meat doesn't need to be the main ingredient. We'd rather eat slightly less and pay a little more for meat from animals that have lived a good life.

serves 4

400–600 g sirloin steak (or fillet
    of beef, silverside)
1 bunch rocket, rinsed
½ tsp salt
2 tbsp olive oil
3 tbsp roasted pine nuts
2 tbsp grated Parmesan
salt and pepper for seasoning

1. Cut the meat into 1 cm cubes.
2. Grind the rocket, salt and olive oil using a mortar and pestle.
3. Mix with the meat and season with salt and black pepper.
4. Toast the pine nuts in a dry frying pan.
5. Top with roasted pine nuts and Parmesan.

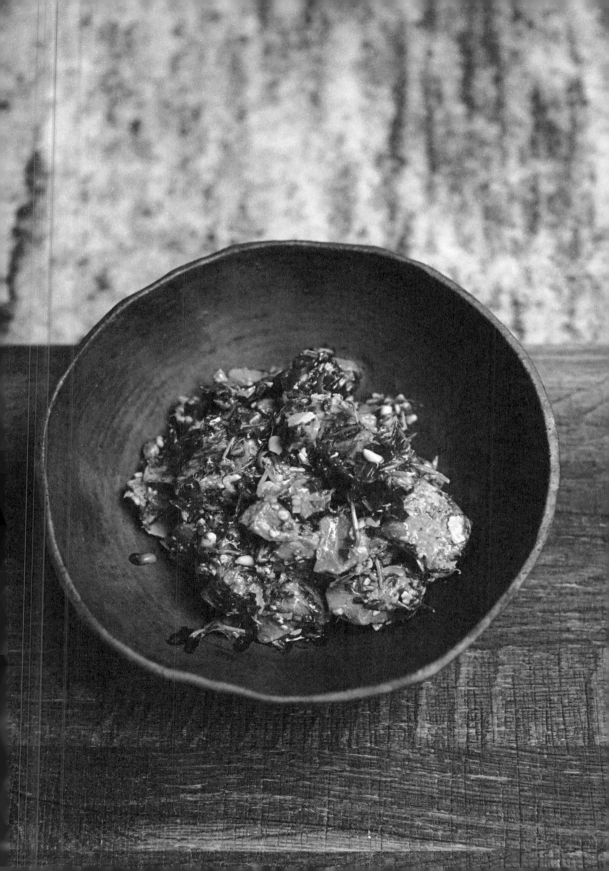

ALL IN ONE

(but not in a blender)

CHAPTER 14.

Change your gut flora in 24 hours

How do you feel? Full of new knowledge and perhaps slightly confused? Relax. It's not that difficult really. A lot of the knowledge recent research has discovered about food are things our ancestors did completely unconsciously.

What is new is that research has caught up and that we can now demonstrate scientifically how the things we eat affect our gut – and our well-being.

We're at the end of the beginning of a development that leads straight towards a future where we will be able to optimise our own food and health based on our own individual needs. In the past people lived for many generations in the same place and their gut flora could be developed in perfect harmony with the food that grew there.

Today, both we and the food we eat move all over the planet. Without even being conscious of it, this means we have cut the 1,000-year link connecting our home environment and our gut flora. Of course it's impossible to go back, so the most likely path ahead of us is to learn to better analyse and understand our own gut flora and how we can eat to be healthiest. The food of the future might well be very local.

We're not quite there yet. But we're on the right road, and as we have seen, it's possible to do something sensible about the situation straight away.

We now know that it's possible to change our gut flora with the food we eat, and that it can be a quick process – measurable changes take place within 24 hours.

A new generation of bacteria is born in your gut about every 20 minutes, and within 10 hours a single bacterium can have given rise to a billion more. Every time we eat something we give a boost to the particular gut bacteria – whether good or bad – that live on breaking down that type of food. Just a couple of hours after the fibre has reached the colon, the fermentation process has begun.

Within seven days you can make your vast gut flora completely change direction – from being dominated by bacteria that live on a typical Western animal-based diet (Bacteroides) to other strains that survive on a vegetarian diet (Prevotella).

Forget everything you have learned about it taking decades before lifestyles and eating habits have an effect! Or that everyone has to eat in the same way. Research into our gut bacteria reveals that we are able to adapt very quickly. The result is a gut flora in constant change. But also that you can both improve and impair your health almost in real time.

The perfect happy salad

There are still many unanswered questions, but some things we know. The more types of gut bacteria you have, the more stable your gut flora – and the better you'll feel!

The important message to remember is simply this: don't eat a boring diet. Eat lots of different foods! This means that you consume different types of fibre, giving the biggest chance that all of your bacteria will continue to be happy and friendly and will want to stay.

And another important tip: Try not to exclude any ingredient completely!

We used to say "eat fruit and vegetables." Ideally leafy green vegetables!

Today we know that we can be slightly more accurate. We have drawn up a check list that you can use to make a salad that's perfect, not just for you, but also for your microbes.

Basic ingredients — include something from each group:

Legumes: kidney beans, black beans, common beans, mung beans or other beans; yellow and green peas, chickpeas, lentils.

Whole grain (boiled, whole or coarsely chopped):
barley, oats, rye, buckwheat, millet, quinoa, brown rice, teff, popcorn. NB! You should ideally vary between barley, oats and rye, as they each contain different types of fibre.

Cruciferous vegetables:
broccoli, kale, pak choi, Brussels sprouts, cauliflower, red cabbage, horseradish, radishes, turnip, watercress.

Leafy green vegetables:
spinach, chard, rocket, nettles, dandelions.

Alliums:
garlic, spring onions, red onion, yellow onion. These are good sources of inulin. Vary with Jerusalem artichokes or green bananas if you like.

Topping:

Olive oil:
If you prefer another fat, choose one that's as fresh and little processed as possible, regardless of whether it's animal or plant-based. Reduce oils with lots of omega-6, and completely avoid hydrogenated fats.

Seeds and nuts:
walnuts, Brazil nuts, cashew nuts, almonds, hazelnuts, pistachios, macadamia nuts, peanuts (actually a legume), pumpkin seeds, sunflower seeds, sesame seeds, chia seeds.

Vary with:

Berries (fresh, dried or frozen):
lingonberries, blueberries, blackberries, goji berries, red grapes, strawberries, raspberries, currants, cherries.

Fruit:
apples, bananas, melon, avocados, pineapple, oranges, figs, dates, plums, pomegranate, mangoes, kiwi.

Herbs and spices:
turmeric, black pepper, ginger, oregano, basil, mustard powder, thyme, nutmeg, cloves, coriander, cinnamon.

Mushrooms:
chestnut mushrooms, shiitake, oyster mushrooms, chanterelles, Pleurotus eryngii (king trumpet mushrooms) and Grifola frondosa (hen of the woods), enokitake.

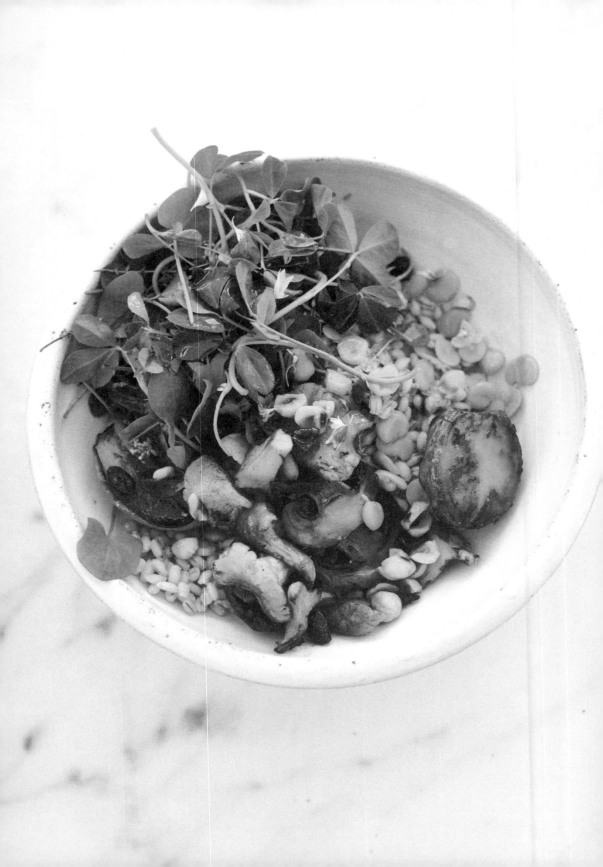

Super salad with beans, barley, Jerusalem artichoke and apple

Different gut bacteria like different things, so if you eat a repetitive diet your gut flora will be equally one-sided. Here is a salad that contains a wide range of different fibre types, so that all your bacterial dinner guests get something they like.

serves 4

6–10 Jerusalem artichokes
8–12 mushrooms
1 bunch thyme
5 tbsp olive oil
1 apple
100 g cooked black beans
100 g cooked whole barley
2 tbsp red wine vinegar
100 g broad beans
100 g hazelnuts, roasted
2 tbsp dried cranberries
salt and freshly ground black
    pepper to season

1. Preheat the oven to 180°C.
2. Wash the Jerusalem artichokes and cut lengthways.
3. Cut the mushrooms into wedges.
4. Place the Jerusalem artichokes and mushrooms in an ovenproof dish with the thyme and pour over 2 tbsp olive oil and salt.
5. Place in the oven and cook for 30 minutes or until the Jerusalem artichokes are almost soft in the middle.
6. Cut the apple into wedges and place in the same dish.
7. Continue to roast for 10 minutes.
8. Mix the beans and barley with the vinegar and remaining olive oil. Season with salt and pepper.
9. Top with roasted vegetables, beans, hazelnuts and cranberries.

Super salad with quinoa, pak choi and pineapple

Eat all the colours of the rainbow! It's not just a variation of fibre types that helps you to feel good – you should also make sure your food contains as many colours as possible. The colours represent different groups of healthy substances in the food.

serves 4

2 heads of pak choi
100 g bean sprouts
¼ pineapple
3 cm fresh ginger
3 black peppercorns
1 lemon, squeezed juice
50 ml olive oil
200 g cooked quinoa
1 bunch beetroot leaves (or other
     bitter plant such as rocket)
1–2 turnips, thinly sliced
6–10 macadamia nuts
salt and freshly ground black
     pepper to season

1. Cut the pak choi lengthways and cook in lightly salted water for 30 seconds, then cool in ice water.
2. Cook the bean sprouts for 3–5 seconds in salted water, then cool in ice water.
3. Peel the pineapple and ginger. Blend until smooth in a food processor with the black peppercorns and lemon juice.
4. Continue to blend and add the olive oil a little at a time. Season with a little salt and more ginger and black pepper if required.
5. Mix the quinoa and pineapple and ginger dressing.
6. Top with pak choi, bean sprouts, beetroot leaves, turnip and chopped macadamia nuts.

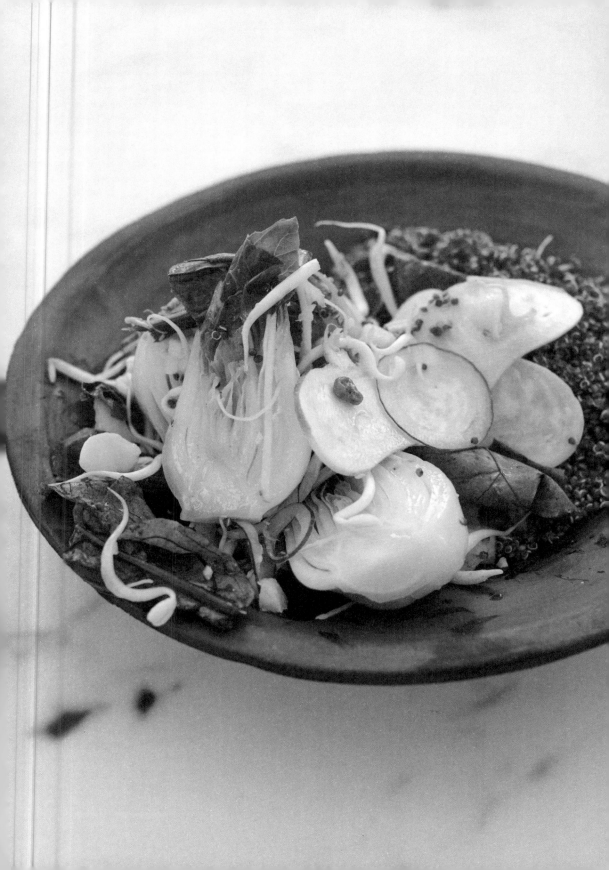

Super salad with lentils, avocado and chard

Vary the flavours! Herbs are full of healthy polyphenols. The food that is the tastiest and smells the best is often also the healthiest.

serves 4

1 bunch chard
200 g cooked lentils
2 spring onions, shredded
2 limes, squeezed juice
4 tbsp olive oil
2 avocados
3 tbsp pistachio kernels
1 bunch watercress

1. Steam the chard for around 1 minute or boil in salted water for 20 seconds.
2. Place the warm chard in a bowl with the lentils and spring onion.
3. Squeeze over the lime juice and drizzle over olive oil.
4. Stone the avocados and slice lengthways.
5. Lay the mixed vegetables on a large dish and top with avocado, pistachio nuts and watercress.

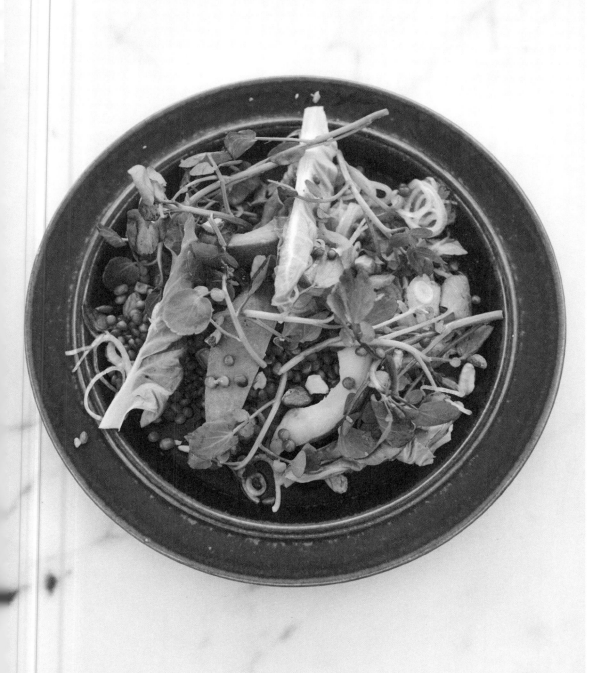

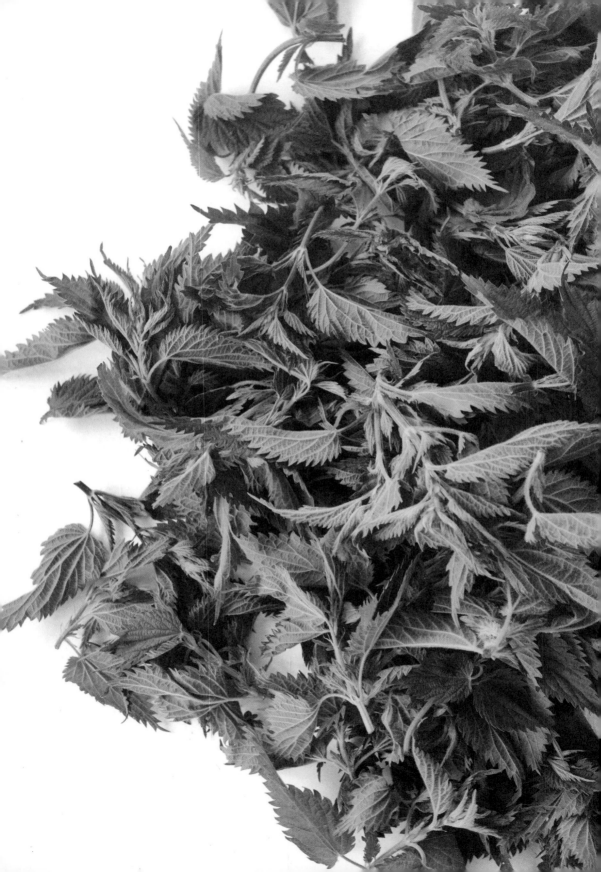

TOP TIP!

Explore your local area!
The most nutritious food can grow wild just around the corner. But get into the habit of washing what you find carefully and don't pick close to busy roads. Only pick things you're sure you can identify.

There are countless edible plants all around us.

Here's a small selection:

Ground elder – use like spinach and chard. Pick early in the spring, and then the new shoots.

Dandelion – add the tender leaves to a salad.

Garlic mustard – use as basil, in a pesto, dressing, herb butter or sprinkle over a salad. Gives a faint garlic flavour.

Grass-leaved orache – grows on beaches, slightly salty taste. Use like spinach and rocket.

Nettle soup

The healthiest food is closer than you think. A tasty, hot nettle soup with shallots and flavoured with a little Pernod and star anise gives you a bowlful of fibre, nitrate and healing polyphenols.

serves 4

200 g nettles
1 shallot
½ tsp fennel seeds
1 tbsp butter
600 ml chicken stock
1 star anise
400 ml Pernod
½ tsp salt

1. Clean and rinse the nettles.
2. Peel the shallot and chop finely.
3. Fry the shallot and fennel seeds in butter without allowing the shallot to brown.
4. Add the stock and star anise and allow to simmer for 15 minutes.
5. Remove the star anise.
6. Increase the heat and add the nettles, bring to the boil and boil for 1 minute.
7. Mix the soup until smooth with a blender.
8. Add the Pernod and season with salt if required.

QUICK START TIPS

In everyday life, it's not always easy to break habits. Here are a few simple tips that have helped us.

Happy 1:

Purge your pantry of happiness thieves that trigger inflammation and depression:

- Sugar
- Finely ground white flour
- Too much alcohol
- Processed convenience foods
- E additives, primarily the flavour enhancer MSG, sweeteners and emulsifiers
- Gluten – if you are sensitive
- Fast carbohydrates such as white unfermented bread, white rice and white pasta
- Palm oil, trans fats and other refined oils
- Chips, margarine, sunflower oil and fried food containing omega-6
- As much as possible, eat food cooked from fresh ingredients

Happy 2:

Every day, eat vegetables that contain a wide variation of fibre types.

Make your own favourite versions of the perfect happy salad. Whole grains (boiled or coarsely chopped), ideally of barley, beans, some kind of onion, leafy green vegetables, other vegetables, olive oil, fruit, nuts and seeds.

Every day eat a little fermented food such as sauerkraut, kefir or perhaps unpasteurised cheese.

Eat all the colours of the rainbow. Make it a habit to include as many colours as possible on your plate. Choose colourful alternatives when you buy food.

Eat tasty, deliciously scented food with a large proportion of aromatic herbs and spices.

Challenge yourself every week by buying at least one vegetable or other ingredient that you don't normally eat!

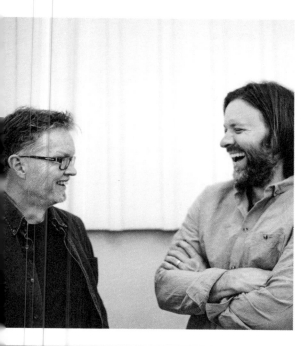

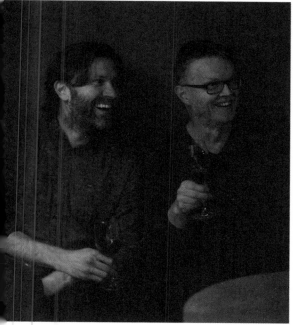

Happy 3:

Don't smoke.

Do plenty of exercise! Provide a more varied gut flora.

Be less stressed! Stress exacerbates the effects of junk food.

Try to stick to a regular circadian rhythm for food and sleep.

Avoid antibacterial detergent, mouthwash, hand cleaner etc.

Get out and meet people. Be physical and touch other people (if they think this is OK).

Ideally, have a dog (but only if you like them!)

Potter in the garden. The soil is rich in bacteria.

But have respect for unfriendly bacteria. Never eat salad – and particularly not onion – which has been chopped several days previously. Be careful with raw chicken, and minced meat which has been prepared a long time in advance.

Good luck!
Henrik & Niklas

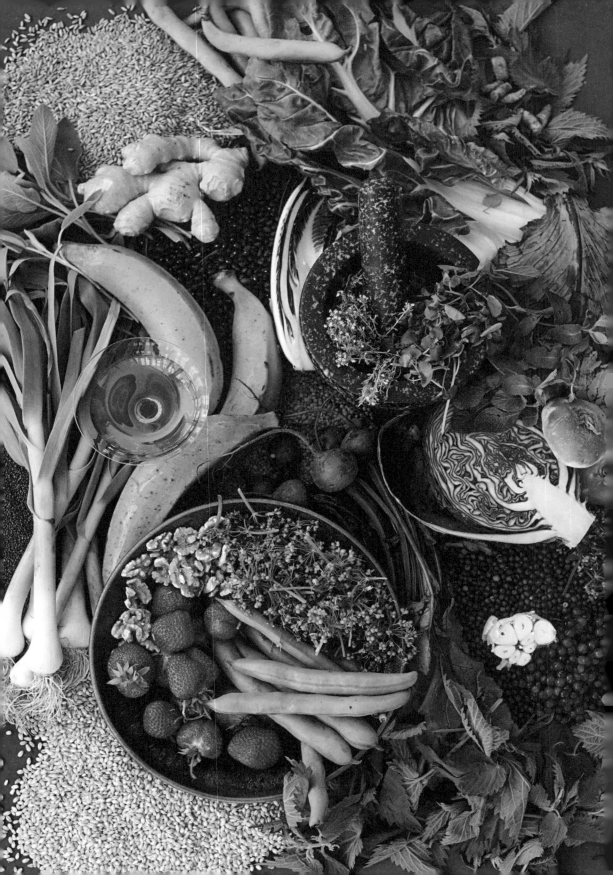

Recipes

Index

Bibliography

Adriana D.T. F, Raymond W. S, Guy A. C. Evaluation of Resistant Starch Content of Cooked Black Beans, Pinto Beans, and Chickpeas. NFS Journal 2016;(C):8–12.

Albenberg L, Wu G. Diet and the Intestinal Microbiome: Associations, Functions, and Implications for Health and Disease. Gastroenterology. 2014;146(6):1564–1572.

Alcock J, Maley C, Aktipis C. Is Eating Behavior Manipulated by the Gastrointestinal Microbiota? Evolutionary Pressures and Potential Mechanisms. Bioessays: News And Reviews In Molecular, Cellular And Development Biology. 2014;36(10):940-949.

Allen A, Dinan T, Clarke G, Cryan J. A Psychology of the Human Brain-Gut-Microbiome Axis. Social and Personality Psychology Compass. 2017;11(4):n/a.

Anderson S, Cryan J. F, Dinan T. The Psychobiotic Revolution: Mood, Food, and the New Science of the Gut-Brain Connection. Publishers Weekly, 2017;264(34):106.

Bailey M, Dowd S, Galley J, Hufnagle A, Allen R, Lyte M. Exposure to a Social Stressor Alters the Structure of the Intestinal Microbiota: Implications for Stressor-induced Immunomodulation. Brain, Behavior, and Immunity, 2011;25:397-407.

Bakker G, van Erk M, Hendriks H, et al. An Anti-inflammatory Dietary Mix Modulates Inflammation and Oxidative and Metabolic Stress in Overweight Men: a Nutrigenomics Approach. The American Journal of Clinical Nutrition, 2010;91(4):1044-1059.

Barrett E, Ross R, O'Toole P, Fitzgerald G, Stanton C. - Aminobutyric Acid Production by Culturable Bacteria from the Human Intestine. Journal of Applied Microbiology, 2012;113(2):411-417.

Benedict C, Vogel H, Cedernaes J, et al. Gut Microbiota and Glucometabolic Alterations in Response to Recurrent Partial Sleep Deprivation in Normal-weight Young Individuals. Molecular Metabolism 2016;5:1175-1186.

Blottière H, de Vos W, Ehrlich S, Doré J. Human Intestinal Metagenomics: State of the Art and Future. Current Opinion in Microbiology 2013;16(3):232 -239.

Bourassa M, Alim I, Bultman S, Ratan R. Butyrate, Neuroepigenetics and the Gut Microbiome: Can a High Fiber Diet Improve Brain Health? Neuroscience Letters 2016;625:56-63.

Bowtell J. L, Aboo-Bakkar Z, Conway M. E, Adlam A. R, Fulford J. Enhanced Task Related Brain Activation and Resting Perfusion in Healthy Older Adults After Chronic Blueberry Supplementation. Applied Physiology, Nutrition, and Metabolism 2017;42(7):773-779.

Campbell, Kristina. The Well-fed Microbiome Cookbook: Vital Microbiome Diet Recipes to Repair and Renew the Body and Brain. Berkeley: Rockridge Press, 2016.

Cani P, Amar J, Burcelin R, et al. Metabolic Endotoxemia Initiates Obesity and Insulin Resistance. Diabetes 2007;56:1761-1772.

Cavicchia P, Steck S, Hébert J, et al. A New Dietary Inflammatory Index Predicts Interval Changes in Serum High-Sensitivity C-Reactive Protein. Journal of Nutrition 2009;139(12):2365-2372.

Cerdá B, Pérez M, Pérez-Santiago J. D, et al. Gut Microbiota Modification: Another Piece in the Puzzle of the Benefits of Physical Exercise in Health? Front Physiol 2016;7:51.

Chassaing B, Koren O, Gewirtz A, et al. Dietary Emulsifiers Impact the Mouse Gut Microbiota Promoting Colitis and Metabolic Syndrome. Nature 2015;519(7541):92-96.

Chopan M, Littenberg B. The Association of Hot Red Chili Pepper Consumption and Mortality: A Large Population-Based Cohort Study. PLOS One, 2017.

Claesson M, Jeffery I, O'Toole P, et al. Gut Microbiota Composition Correlates with Diet and Health in the Elderly. Nature 2012;488(7410):178-184.

Cohen S, Janicki-Deverts D, Turner R. B, et al. Chronic Stress, Glucocorticoid Receptor Resistance, Inflammation, and Disease Risk. Proceedings of the National Academy of Sciences of the United States of America 2012;(16):5995.

Costa R, Snipe R, Kitic C, Gibson P. Systematic Review: Exercise-induced Gastrointestinal Syndrome—Implications for Health and Intestinal Disease. Alimentary Pharmacology & Therapeutics 2017;46(3):246-265.

Crumeyrolle-Arias M, Jaglin M, Rabot S, et al. Absence of the Gut Microbiota Enhances Anxiety-like Behavior and Neuroendocrine Response to Acute Stress in Rats. Psychoneuroendocrinology 2014;42:207–217.

Cryan J, Dinan T. Mind-altering Microorganisms: the Impact of the Gut Microbiota on Brain and Behaviour. Nature Reviews. Neuroscience 2012;13(10):701-712.

Curry B. H, Bond V, Millis R, et al. Effects of a Dietary Beetroot Juice Treatment on Systemic and Cerebral Haemodynamics – A Pilot Study. Journal of Clinical & Diagnostic Research 2016;10(7):1-5.

David L, Maurice C, Turnbaugh P, et al. Diet Rapidly and Reproducibly Alters the Human Gut Microbiome. Nature 2014;505(7484):559-563.

De Filippo C, Cavalieri D, Hartl D. L, et al. Impact of Diet in Shaping Gut Microbiota Revealed by a Comparative Study in Children from Europe and Rural Africa. Proceedings of the National Academy of Sciences of the United States of America 2010;107(33):14691–14696.

de Mello V. D, Paananen J, Lindstrom J, et al. Indolepropionic Acid and Novel Lipid Metabolites are Associated with a Lower Risk of Type 2 Diabetes in the Finnish Diabetes Prevention Study. Scientific Reports 2017.

De Palma G, Collins S, Berick P, Verdu E. The Microbiota-gut-brain Axis in Gastrointestinal Disorders: Stressed Bugs, Stressed Brain or Both? The Journal of Physiology 2014;592(14):2989-2997.

De Vadder F, Kovatcheva-Datchary P, Martens E, et al. Dietary Fiber-Induced Improvement in Glucose Metabolism Is Associated with Increased Abundance of Prevotella. Cell Metabolism 2015;22(6):971-982.

Desbonnet L, Garrett L, Clarke G, Kiely B, Cryan J, Dinan T. Effects of the Probiotic Bifidobacterium Infantis in the Maternal Separation Model. Neuroscience 2010;170(4):1179-1188.

Dimitrov S, Hulteng E, Hong S. Inflammation and Exercise: Inhibition of Monocytic Intracellular TNF Production by Acute Exercise via ß2-adrenergic Activation. Brain, Behavior & Immunity 2017;61:60-68.

Dinan T, Stilling R, Stanton C, Cryan J. Collective Unconscious: How Gut Microbes Shape Human Behavior. Journal of Psychiatric Research 2015;63:1-9.

EFSA CONTAM Panel. Scientific Opinion on the Risks for Human Health Related to the Presence of 3- and 2-monochloropropanediol (MCPD), and their fatty acid esters, and glycidyl fatty acid esters in food. EFSA Journal 2016;15(5).

Engels C, Ruscheweyh H, Beerenwinkel N, Lacroix C, Schwab C. The Common Gut Microbe Eubacterium Hallii also Contributes to Intestinal Propionate Formation. Frontiers in Microbiology 2016;7:713.

Federici E, Prete R, Lazzi, C, et al. Bacterial Composition, Genotoxicity, and Cytotoxicity of Fecal Samples from Individuals Consuming Omnivorous or Vegetarian Diets. Frontiers in Microbiology 2017;8:300.

Fedintsev A, Kudryavtseva A, Baranova A, et al. Markers of Arterial Health Could Serve as Accurate Non-invasive Predictors of Human Biological and Chronological Age. Aging 2017;9(4):1280—1292.

Fernandez-Real J, Ricart W, Portero-Otin M, et al. Gut Microbiota Interacts with Brain Microstructure and Function. Journal of Clinical Endocrinology And Metabolism 2015;100(12):4505-4513.

Finegold S. M, Liu C, Dixon D, et al. Pyrosequencing Study of Fecal Microflora of Autistic and Control Children. Anaerobe 2010;16(4):444-453.

Fujimura K, Demoor T, Lynch S, et al. House Dust Exposure Mediates Gut Microbiome Lactobacillus Enrichment and Airway Immune Defense Against Allergens and Virus Infection. Proceedings of the National Academy of Sciences of the United States of America 2014;111(2):805-810.

Golubeva A. V, Desbonnet L, Zhdanov A, et al. Prenatal Stress-induced Alterations in Major Physiological Systems Correlate with Gut Microbiota Composition in Adulthood. Psychoneuroendocrinology 2015;60:58-74.

Grenham S, Clarke G, Cryan J, Dinan T. Brain-gut-microbe Communication in Health and Disease. Frontiers in Physiology 2011;2:94.

Grootaert C, Van den Abbeele P, Van de Wiele T, et al. Comparison of Prebiotic Effects of Arabinoxylan Oligosaccharides and Inulin in a Simulator of the Human Intestinal Microbial Ecosystem. FEMS Microbiology Ecology 2009;69(2):231-242.

Guyenet, Stephan J. The hungry brain: Outsmarting the instincts that makes us overeat. New York: Flatiron Books, 2017.

Han B, Sivaramakrishnan P, Wang M, et al. Microbial Genetic Composition Tunes Host Longevity. Cell, 2017;169(7):1249-1262.

Head R, Zabaras D, Ooi L, et al. Anti-inflammatory Effects of Five Commercially Available Mushroom Species Determined in Lipopolysaccharide and Interferon-gamma Activated Murine Macrophages. Food Chemistry 2014;148:92-96.

Herieka M, Faraj T, Erridge C. Reduced Dietary Intake of Pro-inflammatory Toll-like Receptor Stimulants Favourably Modifies Markers of Cardiometabolic Risk in Healthy Men. Nutrition, Metabolism and Cardiovascular Diseases 2016;26(3):194-200.

Hesselmar B, Sjöberg F, Saalman R, et al. Pacifier Cleaning Practices and Risk of Allergy Development. Pediatrics 2013;(6):1829.

Hsiao E. Y, McBride S, Mazmanian S, et al. Microbiota Modulate Behavioral and Physiological Abnormalities Associated with Neurodevelopmental Disorders. Cell 2013;155(7):1451-1463.

Huffnagle G. B, Noverr M. The Emerging World of the Fungal Microbiome. Trends Microbiol 2013;21(7):334-341.

Jacka F. N, Cherbuin N, Anstey K, Sachdev P, Butterworth P. Western Diet is Associated with a Smaller Hippocampus: a Longitudinal Investigation. BMC Medicine 2015;13(1):1-8.

Johansson E, Nilsson A, Östman E, Björck I. Effects of Indigestible Carbohydrates in Barley on Glucose Metabolism, Appetite and Voluntary Food Intake Over 16 h in Healthy Adults. Nutrition Journal 2013;12:46.

Johansson, Martina. Hormonbibeln: Hormon-optimering för den moderna människan. Stockholm: Pagina, 2014.

Kamada N, Chen G, Inohara N, Núñez G. Control of Pathogens and Pathobionts by the Gut Microbiota. Nature Immunology 2013;14(7): 685–690.

Karl J. P, Margolis L, Kumar R, et al. Changes in Intestinal Microbiota Composition and Metabolism Coincide with Increased Intestinal Permeability in Young Adults Under Prolonged Physiologic Stress. American Journal Of Physiology - Gastrointestinal And Liver Physiology 2017;312(6):559–571.

Khalid S, Barfoot K. L, May G, et al. Effects of Acute Blueberry Flavonoids on Mood in Children and Young Adults. Nutrients 2017;9(2):158.

Knight R, Cryan J, Mayer E. A, et al. Gut Microbes and the Brain: Paradigm Shift in Neuroscience. Journal of Neuroscience 2014;34(46):15490-15496.

Lai J. S, Hure A, Hiles S, McEvoy M, Attia J, Bisquera A. A Systematic Review and Meta-analysis of Dietary Patterns and Depression in Community-dwelling adults. American Journal of Clinical Nutrition 2014;99(1):181-197.

Larsen F, Ekblom B, Sahlin K, Weitzberg E, Lundberg J. Effects of Dietary Nitrate on Blood Pressure in Healthy Volunteers. New England Journal of Medicine 2006;355(26):2792-2793.

Le Chatelier E, Prifti E, Mérieux A, et al. Richness of Human Gut Microbiome Correlates with Metabolic Markers. Nature 2013;500(7464):541-546.

Leitão-Gonçalves R, Carvalho-Santos Z, Ribeiro C, et al. Commensal Bacteria and Essential Amino Acids Control Food Choice Behavior and Reproduction. PLoS Biology 2017;15(4):1-29.

Li Y, Lv M, Li B, et al. Dietary Patterns and Depression Risk: A meta-analysis. Psychiatry Research 2017;253:373-382.

Liu B, Fang F, Chen H, et al. Vagotomy and Parkinson Disease: A Swedish Register-based Matched-cohort Study. Neurology 2017;88(21):1996-2002.

López-González Á, Grases F, Perelló J, et al. Protective Effect of Myo-inositol Hexaphosphate (Phytate) on Bone Mass Loss in Postmenopausal Women. European Journal of Nutrition 2013;52(2):717-726.

Louveau A, Smirnov I, Kipnis J, et al. Structural and Functional Features of Central Nervous System Lymphatic Vessels. Nature, 2015;523(7560):337-341.

Lozupone C. A, Stombaugh J, Gordon J, Jansson J, Knight R. Diversity, Stability and Resilience of the Human Gut Microbiota. Nature 2012;489(7415):220-230.

Luczynski P, McVey Neufeld K, Oriach C, Clarke G, Dinan T, Cryan J. Growing up in a Bubble: Using Germ-free Animals to Assess the Influence of the Gut Microbiota on Brain and Behaviour. International Journal of Neuropsychopharmacology 2016;19(8).

Lv W, Christophersen C, Sorich M, Gerber J, Angley M, Conlon M. Increased Abundance of Sutterella spp. and Ruminococcus Torques in Feces of Children with Autism Spectrum Disorder. Molecular Autism 2013;4(1):1-7.

Lyte M. Microbial Endocrinology in the Microbiome-gut-brain Axis: How Bacterial Production and Utilization of Neurochemicals Influence Behavior. Plos Pathogens 2013;9(11).

Mammen G, Faulkner G. Review and Special Articles: Physical Activity and the Prevention of Depression: a Systematic Review of Prospective Studies. American Journal of Preventive medicines 2013;45(5):649-657.

Mariat D, Firmesse O, Furet J, et al. The Firmicutes/Bacteroidetes Ratio of the Human Microbiota Changes with Age. BMC Microbiology 2009;9(1):123.

Matsumoto T, Kimura T, Hayashi T. Aromatic Effects of a Japanese Citrus Fruit—Yuzu (Citrus junos Sieb. ex Tanaka)—on Psychoemotional States and Autonomic Nervous System Activity During the Menstrual Cycle: a Single-blind Randomized Controlled Crossover Study. Biopsychosocial Medicine 2016;10.

Matsumura K, Noguchi H, Nishi D, Hamazaki T, Matsuoka Y. Effects of Omega-3 Polyunsaturated Fatty Acids on Psychophysiological Symptoms of Post-traumatic Stress Disorder in Accident Survivors: A Randomized, Double-blind, Placebo-controlled Trial. Journal of Affective Disorders 2016.

McKean J, Naug H, Nikbakht E, Amiet B, Colson N. Probiotics and Subclinical Psychological Symptoms in Healthy Participants: A Systematic Review and Meta-Analysis. Journal of Alternative & Complementary Medicine 2017;23(4):249-258.

Montiel-Castro A.. J, González-Cervantes R. M, Bravo-Ruiseco G, Pacheco-Lopez G.The Microbiota–gut–brain Axis: Neurobehavioral Correlates, Health and Sociality. Frontiers in Integrative Neuroscience 2013;7.

Nehlig A. The Neuroprotective Effects of Cocoa Flavanol and its Influence on Cognitive Performance. British Journal of Clinical Pharmacology 2013;75(3):716-727.

Nicolucci A. C, Hume M, Martinez I, Mayengbam S, Walter J, Reimer R. Prebiotic Reduces Body Fat and Alters Intestinal Microbiota in Children who are Overweight or with Obesity. Gastroenterology 2017;153(3):711-722.

Nilsson A, Johansson E, Ekström L, Björck I. Effects of a Brown Beans Evening Meal on Metabolic Risk Markers and Appetite Regulating Hormones at a Subsequent Standardized Breakfast: A Randomized Cross-Over Study. Plos One 2013;8(4):e59985.

Nilsson A, Ostman E, Holst J, Björck I. Including Indigestible Carbohydrates in the Evening Meal of Healthy Subjects Improves Glucose Tolerance, Lowers Inflammatory Markers, and Increases Satiety after a Subsequent Standardized Breakfast. Journal of Nutrition 2008;138(4):732-739

Nilsson A, Johansson-Boll E, Björck I. Increased Gut Hormones and Insulin Sensitivity Index Following a 3-d Intervention with a Barley Kernel-based Product: a Randomised Cross-over Study in Healthy Middle-aged Subjects. The British Journal of Nutrition 2015;114(6):899-907.

Nurk E, Refsum H, Smith A. Plasma Total Homocysteine and Memory in the Elderly: The Hordaland Homocysteine Study. Annals of Neurology 2005;58(6):847-857.

Nurk E, Drevon C, Smith A, et al. Cognitive Performance Among the Elderly and Dietary Fish Intake: the Hordaland Health Study. The American Journal of Clinical Nutrition 2007;86(5):1470-1478.

Nurk E, Refsum H, Smith A, et al. Intake of Flavonoid-rich Wine, Tea, and Chocolate by Elderly Men and Women is Associated with Better Cognitive Test Performance. Journal of Nutrition 2009;139(1):120-127.

Nurk E, Refsum H, Smith A, et al. Cognitive Performance Among the Elderly in Relation to the Intake of Plant Foods. The Hordaland Health Study. The British Journal of Nutrition 2010;104(8):1190-1201.

Litsfeldt Lars-Erik & Olsson, Patrik. Låt bönor förändra ditt liv. Stockholm: Bladh by Bladh, 2017.

O'Mahony S. M, Clarke G, Borre Y, Dinan T, Cryan J. Serotonin, Tryptophan Metabolism and the Brain-gut-microbiome Axis. Behavioural Brain Research 2015;277:32-48.

O'Neil A, Quirk S, Jacka F, et al. Relationship Between Diet and Mental Health in Children and Adolescents: A Systematic Review. American Journal of Public Health 2014;104(10):e31-e42.

Orlich MJ, Singh PN, Sabaté J, et al. Vegetarian Dietary Patterns and the Risk of Colorectal Cancers. JAMA Internal Medicine 2015;175(5):767-776.

Panduro A, Rivera-Iñiguez I, Sepulveda-Villegas M, Roman S. Genes, Emotions and Gut Microbiota: The Next Frontier for the Gastroenterologist. World Journal of Gastroenterology 2017;23(17):3030-3042.

Pannaraj P. S, Li F, Cerini C, et al. Association Between Breast Milk Bacterial Communities and Establishment and Development of the Infant Gut Microbiome. JAMA Pediatrics 2017;171(7):647-654.

Pérez-López U, Pinzino C, Quartacci M. F, Ranieri A, Sgherri C. Phenolic Composition and Related Antioxidant Properties in Differently Colored Lettuces: A Study by Electron Paramagnetic Resonance (EPR) Kinetics. Journal of Agricultural and Food Chemistry 2014;62(49):12001-12007.

Perry E, Howes M. Medicinal Plants and Dementia Therapy - Herbal Hopes for Brain Aging?, CNS Neuroscience & Therapeutics 2011;17(6):683–698.

Prescott, Susan L & Logan, Alan C. The secret life of your microbiome. Gabriola Island: New Society Publishers, 2017.

Psaltopoulou T, Sergentanis T, Panagiotakos D, Sergentanis I, Kosti R, Scarmeas N. Mediterranean Diet, Stroke, Cognitive Impairment, and Depression: A meta-analysis. Annals of Neurology 2013;74(4):580-591.

Qin J, Li R, Xie Y, et al. A Human Gut Microbial Gene Catalogue Established by Metagenomic Sequencing. Nature 2010;464(7285):59-65.

Opie R, O'Neil A, Jacka F, Pizzinga J, Itsiopoulos C. A Modified Mediterranean Dietary Intervention for Adults with Major Depression: Dietary Protocol and Feasibility Data from the SMILES Trial. Nutritional Neuroscience 2017:1–15.

Rastmanesh R. High Polyphenol, Low Probiotic Diet for Weight Loss Because of Intestinal Microbiota Interaction. Chemico-Biological Interactions 2011;189(1-2):1-8.

Ríos-Covián D, Ruas-Madiedo P, Margolles A, Gueimonde M, De Los Reyes-Gavilan C. G, Salazar N. Intestinal Short Chain Fatty Acids and their Link with Diet and Human Health. Frontiers in Microbiology 2016;7:185.

Sánchez-Villegas A, Martínez-González M, Serra-Majem L, et al. Mediterranean Dietary Pattern and Depression: the PREDIMED Randomized Trial. BMC Medicine 2013;11(1):1-12.

Sarris J, Logan AC, Akbaraly TN, et al. Nutritional Medicine as Mainstream in Psychiatry. Lancet Psychiatry 2015;2(3):271-274.

Sasselli V, Pachnis V, Burns A. The Enteric Nervous System. Developmental Biology 2012;366(1), 64-73.

Schlemmer U, Frølich W, Prieto R, Grases F. Phytate in Foods and Significance for Humans: Food Sources, Intake, Processing, Bioavailability, Protective Role and Analysis. Molecular Nutrition & Food Research 2009;53:330-375.

Sender R, Fuchs S, Milo R. Revised Estimates for the Number of Human and Bacteria Cells in the Body. PloS Biology 2016;14(8):e1002533.

Shetty SA, Hugenholtz F, Lahti L, Smidt H, de Vos W. Intestinal Microbiome Landscaping: Insight in Community Assemblage and Implications for Microbial Modulation Strategies. FEMS Microbiology Reviews 2017;41(2):182–199.

Shinya, Hiromi. The enzyme factor. San Francisco: Council Oak Books, 2007.

Singh RK, Chang H, Liao W, et al. Influence of Diet on the Gut Microbiome and Implications for Human Health. Journal of Translational Medicine 2017;15(1):73.

Slavin J. Fiber and Prebiotics: Mechanisms and Health Benefits. Nutrients 2013;5(4):1417-1435.

Sonnenburg, Justin & Erica. The Good Gut: Taking Control of Your Weight, Your Mood, and Your Long-term Health. New York: Penguin Press, 2014.

Spector, Tim. The diet myth – The real science behind what we eat. London: Weidenfeld & Nicolson, 2015.

Suez J, Thaiss C, Kolodkin-Gal I, et al. Artificial Sweeteners Induce Glucose Intolerance by Altering the Gut Microbiota. Nature 2014;514(7521):181-186.

Thaiss CA, Itav S, Elinav E, et al. Persistent Microbiome Alterations Modulate the Rate of Post-dieting Weight Regain. Nature 2016;540:544-551.

Thaiss C. A, Levy M, Shibolet O, et al. Microbiota Diurnal Rhythmicity Programs Host Transcriptome Oscillations. Cell 2016;167(6):1495-1510.

Tieman D, Zhu G, Klee H, et al. A Chemical Genetic Roadmap to Improved Tomato Flavor. Science 2017;355(6323):391-394.

Walker, AW, Ince J, Flint H, et al. Dominant and Diet-responsive Groups of Bacteria Within the Human Colonic Microbiota. ISME Journal: Multidisciplinary Journal of Microbial Ecology 2011;5(2):220-230.

Vallverdú-Queralt A, Regueiro J, Rinaldi Alvarenga J. F, Martinez-Huelamo M, Leal L. N, Lamuela-Raventos R. Characterization of the Phenolic and Antioxidant Profiles of Selected Culinary Herbs and Spices: Caraway, Turmeric, Dill, Marjoram and Nutmeg. Food Science and Technology 2015;35(1):189-195.

Vincenzo M, Ines V, Giovanni M, et al. Exercise Modifies the Gut Microbiota with Positive Health Effects. Oxidative Medicine and Cellular Longevity 2017.

Vlassara H, Cai W, Uribarri J, et al. Protection Against Loss of Innate Defenses in Adulthood by Low Advanced Glycation End Products (AGE) Intake: Role of the Antiinflammatory AGE receptor-1. The Journal of Clinical Endocrinology Metabolism 2009;94(11):4483–4491.

World Gastroenterology Organisation. WGO Handbook on gut microbes. 2014.

Williams BL, Hornig M, Parekh T, Lipkin W. Application of Novel PCR-Based Methods for Detection, Quantitation, and Phylogenetic Characterization of Sutterella Species in Intestinal Biopsy Samples from Children with Autism and Gastrointestinal Disturbances. Mbio 2012;3(1).

Wu, G. D,Chen J, Lewis J. D, et al. Linking Long-Term Dietary Patterns with Gut Microbial Enterotypes. Science 2011;334(6052):105-108.

Yano J, Yu K, Hsiao E, et al. Indigenous Bacteria from the Gut Microbiota Regulate Host Serotonin Biosynthesis. Cell 2015;161(2):264-276.

Yatsunenko T, Rey F, Gordon J, et al. Human Gut Microbiome Viewed Across Age and Geography. Nature 2012;486(7402):222-227.

Ying H, Qinrui L, Angel Belle C. D, Randi J. H. The Gut Microbiota and Autism Spectrum Disorders. Frontiers In Cellular Neuroscience 2017;11.

Young AJ, Marriott B, Hibbeln J, et al. Blood Fatty Acid Changes in Healthy Young Americans in Response to a 10-week Diet that Increased n-3 and Reduced n-6 Fatty Acid Consumption: a Randomised Controlled Trial. The British Journal of Nutrition 2017;117(9):1257-1269.

Zeissig S, Blumberg R. Life at the Beginning: Perturbation of the Microbiota by Antibiotics in Early Life and its Role in Health and Disease. Nature Immunology 2014;15(4):307-310.

Zollbrecht C, Persson A. E. G, Lundberg J. O, Weitzberg E, Carlström M. Nitrite-mediated Reduction of Macrophage NADPH Oxidase Activity is Dependent on Xanthine Oxidoreductase-derived Nitric Oxide but Independent of S-nitrosation, Redox Biology 2016;10:119–127.

ABSOLUTE PRESS
Bloomsbury Publishing Plc
50 Bedford Square, London, WC1B 3DP, UK

BLOOMSBURY, ABSOLUTE PRESS
and the Absolute Press logo are trademarks of
Bloomsbury Publishing Plc

First published in 2017 by Bookmark Förlag, Sweden.
Published by arrangement with Nordin Agency, AB,
Sweden

First published in Great Britain in 2018

Text © Niklas Ekstedt and Henrik Ennart, 2017
Photography © David Loftus, 2017
Illustrations © Katy Kimbell, 2017

Translated by Quarto Translations, 2018

All rights reserved. No part of this publication may
be reproduced or transmitted in any form or by
any means, electronic or mechanical, including
photocopying, recording, or any information storage or
retrieval system, without prior permission in writing
from the publishers

Bloomsbury Publishing Plc does not have any control
over, or responsibility for, any third-party websites
referred to or in this book. All internet addresses given in
this book were correct at the time of going to press. The
author and publisher regret any inconvenience caused if
addresses have changed or sites have ceased to exist, but
can accept no responsibility for any such changes

A catalogue record for this book is available from the
British Library

Library of Congress Cataloguing-in-Publication data has
been applied for

ISBN   HB: 978-1-4729-5998-0

2 4 6 8 10 9 7 5 3 1

Printed and bound in China by R.R. Donnelley

Bloomsbury Publishing Plc makes every effort to ensure
that the papers used in the manufacture of our books
are natural, recyclable products made from wood grown
in well-managed forests. Our manufacturing processes
conform to the environmental regulations of the country
of origin.

To find out more about our authors and books visit
www.bloomsbury.com and sign up for our newsletters